# WORKING MIRACLES OF LOVE

a collection of teachings
by Yogi Amrit Desai

Kripalu Publications, Box 793, Lenox, MA 01240

Library of Congress Catalog Card Number: 85-50126
ISBN: 0-940258-15-3

Printed in the United States of America
by Kripalu Publications
Box 793
Lenox, MA 01240

### Acknowledgements

**Love: A Flight from Addiction to Freedom** was originally published in 1976 by Kripalu Yoga Fellowship. Copyright © 1976.

**Guru and Disciple: A Relationship of Love** was originally published in 1975 by Kripalu Yoga Ashram. Copyright © 1975.

**God Is Energy** was originally published in 1976 by Kripalu Yoga Fellowship. Copyright © 1976.

"Kundalini Yoga Through Shaktipat" is an original article and originally appeared in **Kundalini, Evolution and Enlightenment** by John White.

**Shaktipat Kundalini Yoga: Frequently Asked Questions** was originally published in 1975 by Kripalu Yoga Ashram. Copyright © 1975.

"Instant Cosmic Consciousness?" is reprinted by permission from **Fate** magazine, July 1975. Copyright © 1975.

# Contents

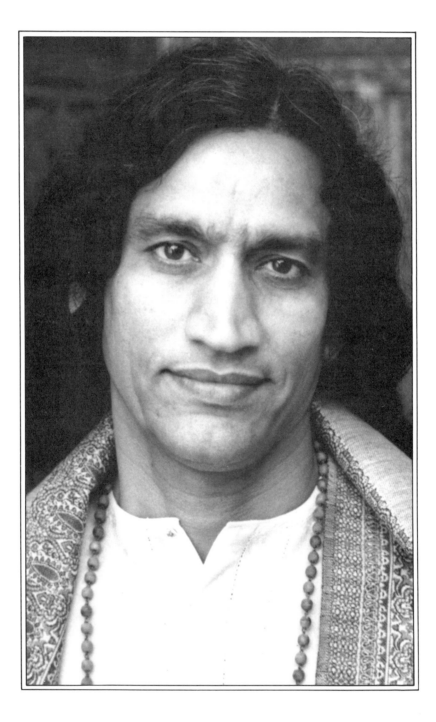

# Introduction

For many years we've separately published the books which are now compiled into this one volume for your convenience.

**Love: A Flight from Addiction to Freedom** gives practical solutions to the problems that we come across daily in our love relationships. It distinguishes true love from attachment, which often comes disguised as love and in fact is the source of our pain and suffering. The discussion also includes the role of sex in loving relationships, the transformation of passion into compassion, and the development of self-love as the foundation for loving others. In the nearly ten years since the book's first printing, thousands of people have gained specific, workable ways to resolve conflicts and create greater harmony and happiness with their co-workers, friends, and family members.

**Guru and Disciple: A Relationship of Love** gives insight into a relationship which is unfamiliar to many Westerners and thus is frequently misunderstood. Rather than presenting an abstract philosophy, this book explains the guru-disciple relationship in practical terms, providing useful guidance for those seeking spiritual growth in daily life.

The book shows that the purpose of this unique relationship is to awaken the "inner guru"—the divine intelligence that dwells within each one of us. It goes on to detail the guru's role as a spiritual teacher, explaining how the guru leads the disciple to non-attachment, self-sufficiency, and higher consciousness. Other topics include the development of trust, faith, and reverence; spiritual disciplines iv and practices; and attunement to the guru's teachings in daily life.

For many people, "God" is an abstract and vague concept, a concept that keeps them from experiencing the truth of their divine nature. **God Is Energy** leads the way to making God a tangible and attainable experience for each of us. This book shows in practical ways how the love of God flows through the body as prana, the vital force of life. It explains how prana can be expressed through the body's seven energy centers, or chakras, which correspond to different levels of consciousness. Using specific methods to raise and balance our energy, we can learn to channel energy through the heart center, expressing prana as love and compassion. The book includes instructions for one such method, the slow motion prana exercise, through which you can experience prana directly as it works in your body.

### Shaktipat Kundalini Yoga

In 1970, Gurudev experienced a great awakening of prana as his whole body entered into a spontaneous flow of yoga postures. This awakening of inner energy is called pranotthana, a preliminary stage of awakening kundalini.

Following this experience, his guru, Swami Kripalvananda, called him to India and gave him shaktipat initiation, a rare blessing bestowed only upon a highly deserving disciple. He gave Gurudev another special blessing at this time: the ability to transfer shakti to others. After Gurudev's own awakening, many people received shakti—the cathartic meditative experiences—in his presence.

As described by D. R. Butler in "Instant Cosmic Consciousness?", people began to experience shakti awakening simply by being in Gurudev's presence. Gurudev wrote **Shaktipat Kundalini Yoga: Frequently Asked Questions** and "Kundalini Yoga Through Shaktipat" in response to many questions people have asked about similar energy experiences. These writings explain how shakti and prana relate to each other, what happens when prana awakens, and how prana functions in the body.

Later Gurudev observed that people who experienced prana awakening often did not have the ability to digest the intensity of their physical, mental, and emotional experiences, so he stopped giving shaktipat. Instead, he incorporated the principles of shaktipat into the new approach to yoga he developed as Kripalu Yoga, which provides the highest benefits of the awakening of prana without its intensity. As a result, everyone can practice and benefit safely.

In kundalini yoga, the mind completely surrenders to prana; prana is allowed complete freedom of expression. In Kripalu Yoga, however, mind and prana work in harmony, the mind remaining a silent yet observant witness.

Understanding the principles of shaktipat leads to understanding how prana works in the body, which is the key to experiencing the full depth and dimension of Kripalu Yoga. Insight into the workings of prana links this modern, holistic approach to yoga with the ancient teachings on the primal, fundamental life energy—the energy which sustains our health, propels the evolution of our consciousness, and works miracles of love in our daily lives.

## Publisher's Note

All text included in this collection appears in its original form and has not been updated or revised for this edition. Therefore, occasional references to people, places, or events which appear outdated are correct with respect to the original time of publication. Current information on Gurudev and Kripalu Center is found on pages 181-184.

# Love: A Flight from Addiction to Freedom

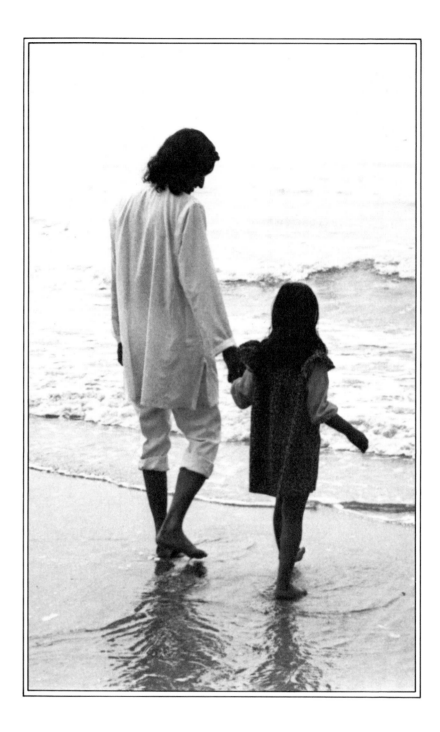

## Love or Addiction: The Plight of Modern Man     3

**Gurudev, the word "love" is used so often today that it has almost lost all meaning. What, according to your definition, is love?**

Love is energy. It is the supreme energy, the highest power that exists. Love is so supreme, so high that man refers to it as God. Love is God, but it is also man's true inner nature. It is the center of man's being for it does not exist apart from him. Man, however, has lost his center. He has acquired the notion that love is to be found outside himself, and so he goes out searching for that which lies within him. He goes begging for that which he already is. He is a king but has mistaken himself to be a beggar.

Because man cannot find love within himself, he seeks a person, an idea, a group which will create in him the feeling of belonging, the feeling of being loved. His search becomes selfish, laden with the desire to find an outside source which will meet his needs. He begins to demand and set up conditions for the other to fill his needs. He wants love, but is willing to give love only when his conditions are met. Such love, based upon conditions, is not love but attachment.

In today's world of self-centered and deteriorating relationships, love has become a very confused and misunderstood concept. Usually what is known as love is no more than attachment. Attachment is a contract, an exchange. "If you do this, I will love you. If you stop doing it, I will no longer love you." Attachment and love are diametrically opposed qualities. They cannot exist simultaneously; they are mutually exclusive. In love, there are no demands, no expectations of the other. You love simply for the sake of loving, for the pure joy of loving in and of itself. In attachment, there are strong expectations. There is a purpose in loving, a desired result, a goal in the relationship and thus the attachment becomes an addiction, a dependence upon

4     receiving the desired goal. When the purpose for the addiction is not fulfilled, you no longer "love".

Attachment focuses on an outside person or object as the center of your being. Love emanates from the center within. Attachment uses the other to fulfill your needs and addictions. The attached person is dependent on the object of his attachment. When the object is gone, the feeling of love is also gone. The person who has contacted his inner source of love, however, carries the light of love with him wherever he goes. He is like a miner with a light attached to his forehead. Wherever he turns, he sees light, because the light is a part of him.

If you truly love, you feel compassion for the other, but you do not make the other the center of fulfillment for your addictions. You are your own center, independent and able to draw happiness from the core of your being. This core becomes the source of all fulfillment for you. As a result, those who come near you receive your freely given gift of love, rather than an exchange of your emotions for their support or acceptance. Such an exchange is not love, but attachment. Attachment is a bargaining process; it is based on sentimentality, the need for control and power and the fear of losing. It ultimately results in pain. Love, on the other hand, expresses itself as compassion, truth, nonviolence, patience, perseverance, tranquility, contentment and joy. It is a factory which produces peace in abundance, the only lasting source of the deep inner happiness man so consistently seeks.

**Why does attachment result in pain? What are the dynamics that lead to that pain and is fear part of that dynamic?**

Attachment begins in fear, lives in fear, dies in fear and is again reborn in fear. Whenever you try to make another person cooperate with you to meet your desires and needs, you are motivated by a selfish purpose. You become dependent on the other to fulfill your needs and consequently, the other's potential absence or lack of cooperation becomes a threat to you. You have created your own threat because you have made the other person the medium to fulfilling your attachment. The more people you objectify as tools to fulfill your attachments, the more entities you are creating, the more individuals you are creating to provide a threat to you. If the person to whom you are attached fails to meet your conditions and expectations, you become even more fearful. This happens because, as you fail to get what you want, you become progressively more afraid of continuously not getting what you want. You become fearful of experiencing the non-fulfillment of your addictions. This fear gives rise to violence, jealousy, competition and hatred, and the person who was at one time the object of your attachment, the object of your fear, now becomes the victim of your fear.

In attachment you love someone in your way. If the other person expects your love to come in a different way, the two "loves" are in conflict. Now you don't have love, but war. The attached person says, "I love you when you meet my needs—in my way. If you do not meet my needs, then I cannot love you. Then you are no good for me." Attachment demands. It specifies particular methods of expression. If the specifications are not met, if the demands are not satisfied, then there is no more love. Love with such conditions is merely a business relationship. It is a bargain. "If you meet my demands, I will love you; if you don't, I won't."

The person with many preferences, with many likes and dislikes, inevitably ends up liking the people who conform to his preferences and hating those who make it difficult for him to get what he wants. As soon as man demands specific conditions, specific people and specific situations to make him happy, he at once labels anyone who acts other than according to his specifications as working against him. He classifies them as enemies and, in this way, he psychologically sets himself apart. In his very act of specifying, he separates himself. Loneliness is the inevitable result.

6    Attachment divides. It is exclusive. Love is all inclusive. It accepts all. It is completely free from fear because it places no demands or conditions on anyone. Attachment creates pain and fear because it wants one thing but not another. Attachment is created out of fear and creates only further fear, but love puts an end to fear.

Because love is universal and unconditional, it is in harmony with all humanity as well as with the forces of nature. Attachment is individual and self-centered. Consequently, it meets conflict everywhere. True love is ultimate adjustability, flexibility and acceptance. Because the person in love is flexible and accepting and is free of expectations, conditions or demands, he has no reason to conflict with any person, situation, belief or disbelief. Conflict is possible only when you experience the other as failing to meet your conditions.

Conditional and selfish love encounters a host of conflicts, resulting in loneliness and fear. To resolve the conflicts resulting from attachment, the attached person feels he needs to fight—to compete for what he wants and prove that he is right. This fight is a fight against a shadow—a shadow created by his own demands and expectations of what should be. As soon as man becomes selfish, he creates his own personal war with the world. The odds in this war are all against him, because he can never make the whole world conform to his specifications. Because attachment generally results in fear and pain, it is a most destructive way to "love" someone.

Love is love forever, but attachment frequently becomes hatred. Love is lasting because it is void of all specifications. All phenomena in the universe exist without specification. Specification is a product of the human mind, created to fulfill individual attachments. Since the mind is limited by time and space, the attachments are also limited by time and space. Thus, in a relationship based on attachment or addiction, as soon as the purpose for the addiction is fulfilled, the love disappears. As long as a person who is attached to another thinks he is going to get what he wants, he remains addicted. As soon as he discovers, however, that he has no possibility of meeting the needs which created the attachment, he ends the relationship. The so-called love collapses. Where there was once love, there now exists only resentment, bitterness, jealousy and competition.

Love is not limited in this way. It has no end. It is not a mental, emotional or egotistical phenomena which is trapped in space and time. It is a universal phenomena, and the person who loves purely is a universal personality. He has merged with existence. He has merged with God, because God is love—timeless, limitless love.

The more sensitive and aware man becomes, the more complete he feels in and of himself. The less he seeks to fulfill his personal needs through other people, situations and the world outside himself, the more he finds fulfillment in himself. He becomes his own center. The whole universe radiates from within such a person. He is in complete mastery of himself. He experiences what yogis describe by saying, "I am that I am"—the state of total contentment and peace. He accepts all—as it is. He accepts himself as he is. He accepts others as they are. In a sense, he becomes free from all the happenings of the phenomenal world, because no happening ever upsets him. He becomes like a lotus in a pond as described in the **Bhagavad Gita** (an ancient yogic scripture). Although the lotus grows in the water, it is never touched by the water. Such a person is in the state of stithapragnia—beyond all duality of success and failure, happiness or unhappiness. Such a person is free of addiction.

When a man feels capable, creative and free, then he can love. When he feels incomplete in himself, he looks for someone who will provide the qualities he lacks. He becomes attached to the person whom he thinks will make him complete. Now he needs the other. He is in bondage to the other. Realizing this subconsciously, he fears the other's withdrawal. Gradually and subtly he begins to hate the

8    other. He cannot help but hate that which is a source of fear and anxiety to him. Even though he himself created the fear and addiction, he paradoxically hates the other as the cause of his insecurities.

Whenever man expects or craves love from another, he unknowingly asks for exactly the opposite of what he wants. Seeking love from the other automatically puts man in bondage to the other. Conversely, when man makes someone dependent upon him or addicted to him, hate is also the result. The person who needs him cannot love him because of the unconscious threat he represents to that person. All addictions and attachments are potential hate problems. Only when man makes himself and the other free from dependence can there be true love, for love is possible only between two free individuals.

Seeking and longing, even in the name of love, corrupts and distorts love. Seeking of such a nature occurs in the external world. Love, however, is found within. Only when man has searched inside himself to uncover the true source of inner love will he be able to experience genuine love in the external world. Christ taught, "the Kingdom of God is inside you" (Luke 17:21). That Kingdom is the source of love within man himself.

Man's desire to be loved is actually a deep inner desire to give love. If his desire to give love becomes tinged with selfishness, however, then it becomes a desire to take love—a desire based upon the expectations and demands of the ego. Love of this sort becomes a contract of conditions in which man desires to capture love, to control love and to gain power over the other. The struggle for power is an inevitable by-product of attachment. By controlling the other, man attempts to protect himself from being hurt by the other. In this process, however, he generates a tremendous amount of tension: earning power creates tension, holding it creates tension and losing it brings total destruction and despair to the one who has made power his goal in life. Love, on the other hand, brings peace in each phase—it brings peace as it comes, as it exists and as it passes. If there is tension in any one of these stages, there is not love but attachment. Attachment breeds the need for power, which in turn creates dependency upon others because it requires recognition by others. Love fosters freedom from power for it is absolute and self-contained.

Power is artificial but love is natural. That which is natural is easy to maintain. If you make a tight fist you can hold it for only a limited period of time, but if you relax your hand, you can keep it relaxed indefinitely without effort. Power is like the tension of a clenched fist which is difficult to maintain. Love is like a relaxed hand. It is man's natural state.

**Gurudev, I have a pet which I love very much. It doesn't feel like attachment, but yet I wonder if it could be. What about love for animals? Is that kind of love inherently selfless and pure in nature, or is it, too, based on conditions and expectations?**

Your relationship with your pet could, of course, be based on pure love—there is always that possibility. For most people, however, love of all sorts, whether it be for a human being, an object or for an animal, has deteriorated into attachment.

Attachment to another human being is a great source of conflict to the average man, so he seeks a safer outlet for his attachment. Often he finds that outlet in love for an animal which he takes for a pet. Love for animals can, of course, be non-attached as I said to you earlier, however, for many people such love serves as an escape from dealing with people. It serves as a method of avoidance.

Man cannot live alone. He must belong. He has a need to be loved and an even greater need to give love. Because of today's deteriorating human relationships caused by an insensitive, selfish and ego-oriented culture, man seeks to fulfill his need for love through his relationship with a pet. An animal has no requirements other than food, which

10 money can buy. The human relationship of attachment has many requirements which are necessary to fulfill the basic selfish reasons for the attachment. Such a relationship also has many opportunities for conflict—conflict of interest, conflict of expectations. Basically, man does not want to deal with these conflicts. He avoids the possibility of having to accept the other or having to change himself for the other.

I recall an incident which clearly illustrates this point. It took place in the waiting room of a New York airport, where I found myself sitting next to a nicely-dressed, handsome young man. I asked him where he was going and we talked for a while. As the conversation continued, I asked him his profession. He shared that he was a mortician. I asked him, "How did you come to select such a profession?" and his answer was that, in his profession, there was no "backtalk". He had found his solution to the problem of relating to others, to the problem of dealing with resistance, competition, hatred and jealousy. By dealing with the dead, he avoided having human relationships which might cause him pain. Although most people don't choose such a drastic measure to avoid the inevitable conflicts present in attached human relationships, many do find other or similar methods of avoidance.

An animal is a perfect outlet for this avoidance. He is the perfect partner for attachment. In an animal, man has a source of receiving love and an object for giving his own love, yet he still has no one to contend with. There is no fear of the other, for the pet can't hurt him. Dumb animals don't argue. Thus man finds a false substitute for love which does not complain or compete and which will never leave him.

It is interesting to note that, at a time when so many human beings need love, more and more people are buying and putting their love into pets. Often they rationalize their actions by saying that they dislike seeing animals misused or abused. In actuality, however, many are afraid that they will not get what they want from people. The fear comes from their desire to get something from the other.

As a result, dogs and cats are pampered with love and attention, in some cases beyond what is even healthy or natural for them, while human beings grow increasingly unstable in their ability to give and receive love.

**Then, what about one's love for his country or for his religion? Are those also forms of attached love?**

In order to understand love for one's country or one's religion, you must first understand that often such love takes place not in the heart, but in the mind. The head-oriented person says, "I love my nation, my religion." These are abstract terms—terms that exist on only a mental level. Often the person who speaks so much of love for his country is using this "love" as a substitute for his fear. When man loves something as abstract as a country or a religion, he doesn't have to deal with people face to face. Personal interaction is the true test of a person's love. Man finds his escape from facing the realities of human interaction by adopting an abstract love for religion, God or for "humanity". You see, "religion" doesn't approach a man and question him. Humanity doesn't hurt him. The person who loves "humanity" but hates his neighbor is an escapist. As soon as he begins to deal with individuals, he is forced to confront himself. Religion will not come to him and make personal demands of him, but an individual may come and ask, "Why are you doing this to me?" God will not come to him, either, even though He can, because the average man has not opened himself to such a point that he can communicate with God. For the average person, even God is still an abstract term.

Loving something in the abstract is often a disguise for needing security and self-importance. It is based on the fear of being less important than others. Such "love" breeds the feeling of separation. If I am to love my country, I must not love countries other than my own. Division of this sort is not the result of love, but of attachment. Such attachment

12    generates fanaticism.

True love is acceptance and compassion for each human being without distinction. Such love can never be obsessed with one group or belief as opposed to all others. Only the head-oriented person can be a fanatic; the heart-oriented person, the person of love and understanding, encompasses all in his love.

Fanatical love is love in name only. In reality such love is a hide-out, a shelter for weak people who justify their fears in the name of God, patriotism or an ideal. Such a love is a cozy castle of conditions, agreements and definitions which exists for the purpose of security. Everything existing outside the castle walls is a threat and therefore an object of hate. Love that has hate as its counterpart is never love, but a mixture of attachment and hate in which hate plays a predominant role in all actions. Although the fanatic might say that he has love for his group or his belief, his actions are more hate-oriented than love-oriented.

Such codified fanatical "love" has created wars in the name of love. To fight for love is an absurd concept. To fight a war to bring peace is self-contradictory. Love is peace, but the so-called "peace" that causes war is not peace—it is competition. Man fights wars for selfishness, and calls it peace. Can you imagine fighting a war for love? It is impossible. Love exists by itself without resorting to or depending on anything other than itself. It does not demand that external things happen in a certain way in order to have peace. Thus the fanatic who claims to love is instead attached and all his actions emerge from that attachment.

## From Passion to Compassion

**What about the role of sex in love? Is sex an expression of pure love or is it an expression of attachment? How should it be used in one's life?**

Sexual expression is usually, although not always, preceded by sensual attraction. When a boy "falls in love" with 13 a girl, or vice versa, he becomes physically and emotionally attracted to her. She appears to him to be capable of meeting his specific expectations, so his attraction is based on conditions. He says, "I love her. She's the one. If I could get her, my life would be changed. I'd have nothing left to worry about." He sees the object of his love only in terms of his own needs and desires. He does not see the other person as she is, nor does he experience her as a person who also has needs and desires. He expects only to find someone who will make him complete. Such immature love is based on imagination, expectation and addiction. It is doomed to failure.

When the one who is attached gets close to the object of his love, he realizes that she is incapable of fulfilling all of his expectations. Differences begin to emerge. If the physical attraction is sufficiently strong, however, each is willing to drown the differences under the high tide of sensual and emotional stimulation they receive from the other. On the basis of this stimulation, they believe that their love will last forever.

Love is non-aggressive and non-violent. It never pushes or imposes. When two people first fall in love, they pretend that they are not aggressive, even though the end is constantly in mind. Each one pretends to have true love. There is no sex, just play. Gradually, as they get to know each other better, the sex act comes, but only after long and delayed foreplay. Even after the act, the play continues. Once they are married, however, the sex act is direct. The foreplay and afterplay are lost. This is the character of seduction or aggressive passion. An act is always performed with a selfish end in mind. As soon as that end is achieved in and through the sex act, the pretense drops and the absence of true love becomes obvious.

It is at this point that the differences, hidden behind the tide of sexual and emotional attraction, begin to emerge. Attraction begins to evaporate; contradictions rise above the surface of the subsiding tide and the so-called

14    love ends in hate. On their wedding day they were willing to die for each other; now, in the divorce court, they want to kill each other. Many such couples divorce legally; others continue their marital relationship for social status, children, money, power or prestige, but rarely for love.

Sex is not love because sex has conditions. When there is only sex and no love, the partners go directly into the sex act. As soon as the sex act is finished, they fall asleep and sometimes even act as if they have nothing to do with each other. In many cases the couple fights all day, creating a vacuum, a lack of pure love, which they try to fill through sensual and emotional enjoyment. So they come together just for the sex act; then they separate again after the act is over. When love follows the sex act, sex becomes ugly; but when sex follows love, sex becomes beautiful. Whenever the lower impulse follows the higher, the lower becomes transformed into the higher. On the contrary, when the higher follows the lower, the higher becomes transformed into the lower. When love follows sex, both love and sex become momentary, painful and goal-oriented. When sex follows love, sex is transformed into true love beyond the barriers of selfish, conditional, aggressive attachments. In other words, the lower does not need to be suppressed; it need only follow the higher. Then it can be transformed and used for higher growth.

The lower forms of attachment and attraction, being emotional, are strong in the initial stages. Such emotional energies are very violent, very obvious and very extroverted. Even a dull person can feel them. They develop very quickly and they deteriorate just as quickly. True love is soft, gentle, non-violent and non-imposing. Great sensitivity is required to feel it, because true love moves like a gentle breeze, a gentle fragrance. People who have become very accustomed to heavy, coarse, violent, aggressive and emotional love are often insensitive to soft, non-attached, true love and compassion. It is so gentle that people who enter the presence of one who truly loves often fail to feel his love. They would feel more if they sat with their girl-friend or boyfriend than if they sat in the presence of the Buddha or of my Gurudev. They would think, "He is just sitting there. He is not even giving a lecture. He is just being silent." And they would feel nothing.

In true love there is no overt excitement or eruption of the emotions. It is difficult for the insensitive person to understand, feel and accept true love, because he is so used to the strong storms of passion and emotion. The compassion of real love is so subtle and so profound that you must feel it to understand it. It takes great sensitivity to learn to understand, accept and respond to true love. As a person grows on the spiritual path, he gradually becomes more aware and more sensitive to such subtle vibrations. He becomes more capable of attuning to the gentle grace, the gentle breeze of love.

**Gurudev, often I feel passionate, I feel like filling that vacuum, as you called it, through emotional or sensual enjoyment. How can I learn to transform that passion into compassion? How can I turn that tendency toward self-enjoyment toward true love for others, not by self-denial, but in a way that will truly fulfill me?**

In order to fully answer your question, I must first explain love and passion as different forms of one energy which exist within the body. This energy is completely neutral in nature. As it flows through the body, it moves through different subtle energy centers called chakras which are located within the spine. Although these chakras do not exist in a physical sense, as do the liver or the kidneys, they do exist in a subtle form in areas corresponding to specific physiological areas.

The chakras in the body are as follows:
**1. Muladhara,** located at the base of the spine
**2. Swadhisthana,** located at the genital region

3. **Manipura,** located at the navel
4. **Anahata,** located at the heart
5. **Vishuddha,** located at the throat
6. **Ajna,** located at the point between the eyebrows
7. **Sahasrara,** located at the crown of the head

The chakras play a crucial role in determining the expression of man's life energy known in yoga as prana. Each center manifests this energy in a particular way. When man's energy is active in a specific chakra, his state of consciousness corresponds to the qualities represented by that chakra. When energy functions in the first chakra, the Muladhara, the qualities of laziness, lethargy, inertia and the drive for security are manifested. A person who acts from the consciousness of the first chakra is in the state or the "guna" known as tamas (inertia). The second chakra, the Swadhisthana, represents sensuality. The person acting from the consciousness of the second chakra is in the state known as rajas (restlessness), the guna characterized by activity. The third chakra represents power and its corresponding guna is also rajas, while the fourth chakra, the Anahata, represents pure love and compassion. The state represented by the fourth chakra is sattva (purity). The fifth chakra, the Vishuddha, represents spontaneous creativity and intuitive wisdom. Its corresponding guna is also sattva. The sixth, the Ajna Chakra, is a bridge between the finite mind and universal consciousness. In the Ajna Chakra, man goes beyond sattva, entering a state of being beyond any mental state of consciousness. From the fourth chakra on, the state known as sattva matures until, in the sixth and seventh chakras, man transcends all three of the basic states or gunas know as tamas, rajas and sattva. In the seventh and uppermost chakra, known as the Sahasrara, man reaches transcendental consciousness or oneness with God, a state of being beyond all duality. He unites with the Brahman in the state described as "one without the other".

The first three chakras are the centers of security,

passion and power. When man's energy is primarily active in these centers, he is ego-oriented. Each of his activities is performed with a desired and selfish goal in mind. All of his relationships, be they personal or of a business nature, are based upon the fulfillment of his conditions, conditions which are designed to serve his desire for security, passion or power. He is aggressive in all aspects of his life. He approaches each situation, each interaction armed with his personal conditions. He sees the world through selfish and ego-oriented eyes, eyes incapable of penetrating the darkness caused by his own passions. His ears hear nothing but the chaos of the clashing forces which exist in the first three levels of consciousness.

The first three chakras are related to the external world. The world within begins with the fourth chakra, the center of the heart. In the fourth chakra, man's energies, which are normally dissipated through passionate and egotistical living, are conserved and transformed into pure and selfless love. It is in this chakra, the chakra of love, that the spiritual journey begins. When man's energy radiates from this chakra, it spreads the divine fragrance of compassion. Now man's value systems are reversed. His consciousness enters an entirely new dimension. The **Bhagavad Gita** describes this process by saying that the yogi is asleep (in the first three chakras) where worldly people are awake, and awake (in the heart chakra) where worldly people are asleep (Chapter 2:69).

When energy is expressed through the second chakra, the sex center, the energy takes on the quality of passion; the same energy expressed through the fourth, or heart center, manifests as compassion. Thus, sexual energy is not bad, it is merely one expression of neutral energy. It is, in fact, most intimately related to the achievement of superconsciousness. Man cannot reach higher states of consciousness without this energy. It is the proper use of sexual energy which determines whether it is harmful or helpful to man, harmful or helpful to his attaining higher states of

18    consciousness and greater peace, love and joy in his life.
      The first three chakras are not, in and of themselves,
of a lower nature. They are merely seats of lower states of
consciousness. They are doors, as are the higher four chakras, through which man's energy expresses itself. Energy
itself is neutral. It is neither positive nor negative. The
reason the first three chakras are called "lower" is simply
because the energy, when allowed to exit through those
doors in search of personal security, sensual gratification
or power, invariably brings destruction, pain and suffering
to man. When man expresses his energy through the lower
three chakras to gratify his passions and ego, he uses his
energy in a way which is harmful to him. The same energy,
when expressed as love and compassion for others, brings
great joy and happiness to him. In other words, when the
first three chakras act as exits and allow energy to dissipate
externally, they are destructive to man. When, however, they
act as passageways to assist the energy in its ascent to the heart
center, they are constructive and fill a divine function.
      Love and aggression, love and passion, love and lust
are diametrically opposed. Energy expressed as aggression,
lust or passion is energy flowing from the first three chakras. Energy expressed as pure love, compassion and creativity is energy flowing from the higher four chakras. When
energy flows from the first three chakras, it is expressed as
aggression, lust and passion. Man is compelled to find an
outlet for this passion through an external person or object. To compensate for the tensions created by this compulsion, he feels the need for greater forms of release from
tension. Then he is further compelled to unburden himself
by dissipating his energies through the sex center.
      The greater man's passion, the greater is his tension;
the greater his passion, the stronger is the force of gravity
which constantly pulls man's consciousness to the lower
chakras. When man uses his energy to love others, he is, in
fact, releasing his energy from the gravity of the lower
chakras. His flood of energy then rises into realms of pure

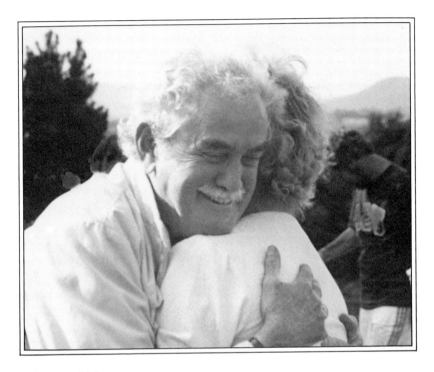

love and bliss.

Man must make a positive effort to curb the energy which is normally drawn downward by the gravitational pull of the lower chakras and to redirect that energy to the heart chakra. The many scientific techniques of yoga are specifically designed to do just this. Ancient yogic techniques act as methods of conserving energy and channeling it into the pure expression of the higher centers. Thus, the regular practice of yoga is a primary and most effective means of transforming passion into compassion.

## The Secrets of Love in Action

**How does a man who has reached the stage of love act? How is his behavior different from that of the person who is attached?**

So few people have reached this state of pure love that

20    it is difficult to describe it in terms the average person can understand. Most people, however, have experienced a lack of love, so perhaps it will be easier to understand what love is by first understanding what love is not.

The person who is not acting from love is the person who cannot accept himself as he is. He is the person who suffers from either an inferiority or a superiority complex. When a person is not objective, when he is one-sided, arrogant or opinionated, he is not acting from love. Hatred, jealousy, anger and competition are diametrically opposed to love, as is any action which is motivated by these negative emotions or by the desire to prove something to someone else. The person who is always motivated by love acts in a very objective manner, disregarding any personal gain or loss that might come to him in any given situation. His emphasis is on helping others rather than on always seeking help. He lets go of the desire to enhance his own image, thereby enhancing his ego, and he never tries to take advantage of another's situation. The man of love acts in direct response to the situation as it is. He has no ulterior motive. He acts in the present according to the present situation. He doesn't bring into play future hopes or past conflicts. As a result, he is fresh in his approach to life. He sees people, situations and ideas as fresh, in the here and now.

When love exists, communication of the highest nature occurs spontaneously. This communication is more like communion—it is a unity which flows from the heart, rather than the head. Attachment does not commune; it tries, instead, to communicate through the mind, through the use of logic and reason. Hatred, jealousy, anger and competition invariably occur when man tries to communicate through a mind which is made subjective by his own motives and desires. A person who cannot communicate with others is not acting from love but from attachment.

The person who acts from love does not act from competition or fear. He does not work for the demon of jealousy. The man who acts from attachment is controlled by his own passion and anger and by his thirst for power. He resorts to manipulating other people and situations because he fears he will lose the objects of his desire. The person who is fearless, who has nothing to lose, because he wants nothing for himself, is the person who acts from love. Such a person is free. His actions are free from tension, impatience and fear because he is not attached to the results of his actions. He accepts what is and what is to be. He lives in the spirit of "Thy will be done, Lord, not mine." Such a person's love is true love.

Love is not saying, "I love you. I love you." Love means giving up all fears and tensions. It means living in harmony with all those around you and all that surrounds you. Love that remains on a verbal or emotional level only is not real love. Real love is action done in love, action done for the good of others. Such actions of love awaken deeper and deeper states of active love.

The greater a person's attachment to people and things, the more burdened he will feel. All objects of attachment assume a great weight because of the ceaseless downward gravitational pull of selfish desires. For the one who is attached, such objects seem to be part of his very person. He identifies with them so strongly that they stick to him like a second skin. Invariably he is forced to be detached from them by circumstances and situations in his life, and then he bleeds the blood of pain and fear. A totally opposite dynamic occurs when a person truly loves. Objects which at one time seemed closely adhered to him suddenly lose their adhesion. Such a person discovers that these things which he at one time identified with are not him at all. In detaching himself from these objects (either literally or emotionally), he finds greater freedom and fulfillment of his being. He begins to gain a deep understanding that all things belong to God—that he didn't bring anything when he came into this world and that he will leave everything behind when he leaves. By consciously choosing to give up what he has and by not wanting things

22 which are not his, he begins to develop an inner trust in God, who dwells within him. He learns to live in attunement to what is, rather than try to maneuver what is to meet his own private, individual sensual or power-oriented needs.

The qualities of real love are highly regarded in the world, as they are essential to its smooth functioning. The business world, for example, cannot function without the pretense of kindness, patience, acceptance and positive attitude toward the customer. Because so few people, however, have actually experienced pure and selfless love, many put on the artificial pretense of love, compassion and understanding in order to be successful. To whatever extent man fakes love, however, he suffers a proportional degree of tension. This tension is the price he pays for pretending to be what he is not.

The business man, for example, must appear to be loving. He must appear to be patient, compassionate and understanding in his dealings with prospective customers. Because his "love" is prompted by an ulterior motive—that of making a sale—and because he has never experienced pure and selfless love, he is forced into pretense. He is required to express the qualities of true love when he simply does not experience true love. He masks his fear, competition or greed beneath a facade of socially-acceptable qualities. If he is a good actor, he succeeds and is accepted by society. He pays a great price for his pretense, however—the price of tension in the form of stomach ulcers, compulsive smoking, drinking and overeating, insomnia, irritability, restlessness, fear and dissatisfaction in his life. Such a man acts from compulsion; compelled by his attachment to possess money, power or prestige, he is also compelled to be other than who he is.

Such a compulsive man gives the control of his life into the hands of another person or into the thing to which he is attached. His addiction inevitably becomes the source of his suffering and self-destruction. Such a man is like the bee that, enchanted by the nectar of the flower, forgets to fly away before the evening when the flower closes—and he dies. In like manner, the snake charmer captures the snake through the very music which enchants the snake. So also, human beings are destroyed through the very things to which they are most attached.

Love can never be compulsive. The flower is not compelled to spread its fragrance. To spread fragrance is its nature. When the lotus of the heart blossoms, it naturally spreads the fragrance of love and compassion to all who come in contact with it. When the true flowering of the heart occurs, the person is not conscious of it, because it is no longer his doing. Love does not occur through his demands, for love is no longer the need or expression of his ego. As lust, passion and the thirst for power are transformed into love, selfless service and surrender, his inner journey begins and soon the fragrance follows wherever he goes. Such a man becomes permeated with the higher qualities of love, magnetism and charisma. His presence has a soothing, healing effect on others. People become transformed in the fragrance of his love, but he is not even conscious of it. They experience in-depth changes in their personalities by just being in his presence, but he himself is doing nothing. He is not even aware of what is happening, why it is happening or how it is happening, for such concerns are the concerns of the ego. When a man reaches this level, his ego has nothing to do with what is happening around him, nor is it fed fat by these occurrences. His love simply happens; it is not done. He has become a hollow channel for the love of God to flow through, a hollow flute through which existence itself plays the melodies of love to touch all who open their hearts to him. He is no longer the doer. Neither the giver nor the receiver of love, he has become love itself. His love is like the sun which shines equally on all, good and bad, rich and poor, healthy and unhealthy, for he has reached a state of pure love energy which is both neutral and all-encompassing in nature. This pure energy is what we call God.

24     Such a love was the love of all the great Masters—of Krishna, Christ and Buddha. Wherever such Masters went, love miracles happened. They were not magicians, but magic itself. The actor in them was absent. They were their actions and their actions were love. They themselves became incarnations of love, sons of the universal, all-pervading God who exists as all-embracing, neutral energy. This energy and its laws are absolute. They exist everywhere. When man transcends his lower nature of self-centered desires, he unites with this pure love energy. He becomes one with God, an enlightened one, a yogi, for the meaning of yoga is union—union of the individual consciousness with the cosmic consciousness of God. Such union is the peak experience of pure love.

**You describe love as gentle and non-aggressive. How does the gentle and loving person acquire enough energy and drive to get along in the world?**

There are two sources of energy: love and ego. The energy of the ego is readily available, but it is very difficult, in the initial stages, to draw energy from love. If you are angry, jealous or competitive, you have tremendous amounts of egotistic energy at your command, but this energy will result in greater degrees of pain and suffering.

To command energy from the ego is much easier than to command energy from love. Egotistical energy is readily available, but it is difficult to get energy from love. The ego provides you with an external playground—with very tangible, solid, familiar satisfaction. You can see the results. You know what you are working with. Love, however, works in a very subtle way. When you work through love, the results are not seen immediately. In the beginning, you have to contend with problems and difficulties without knowing what the results will be. You are working up in the air and for this reason, you will find it easier to work with ego rather than with love. Love means difficulties and ego means immediate satisfaction. Ego satisfaction is immediate, but it sows the seed of inevitable suffering. Love creates some pain in the beginning, but it sows the seed of great joy.

You must experience the ego, however, before you can give it up. Experiencing the ego means suffering. When you get so fat that you cannot even carry your own weight, then you are willing to be put on a fast. Then you are willing to surrender and become light; you are ready to grow wings so you can fly from the cocoon of the ego.

Only after the ego has been reinforced and you are in control can you give it up. When you lack self-identity, the ego is lost, but not out of choice. Once your identity is established, however, you have the choice of giving up the ego. It is an altogether different thing—a very subtle but important point. People who have psychological problems because they have lost their self-confidence, because they have lost their ability to perform ordinary, worldly duties and to function properly, must consciously strengthen the ego. Once their ego is strong, however, they can give it up voluntarily and go back to the same stage where they were involuntarily. The difference lies in the fact that, where previously they were forced into losing the ego, they now can take the step willfully. They are now in control.

The ego is a very real phenomenon, not just a word in a book or the subject of philosophical or psychological studies. The ego actually controls you and your everyday activities. It interferes, intervenes and interprets through each and every action that you perform.

This ego is the total sum of all the impressions that you have received in this lifetime and in previous lifetimes. The central theme of these impressions has been me, mine, you and yours—the theme of individualism and separation. All impressions have been received through this channel of separation and selfishness. Separation and selfishness have built a wall around your divine self, your higher self. Only once in a while does light penetrate through these self-

26 imposed walls. Then you begin to see the glory of the divine self that shines within you, the divine self that is beyond this changing, selfish, ego-self that keeps you forever going in circles on the merry-go-round of life.

Do not consider the ego to be bad. The ego serves an important function. At a certain stage it is good for those who have lost their self-identity to have the ego reinstated. These people are no longer in control of their lives, of their ego. They have to regain control of this ego so they can function normally, because without the ego they feel weak, lost and negative about themselves. They lose all self-confidence.

You must have self-identity. You must have an ego before you can rise above it. The first step is to develop an ego, the second is to relinquish it.

Psychologists agree with this principle and emphasize the importance of the ego. They have one end in mind, however—that of correcting your social behavior so you can accomplish many things and function better in this world. They reinstate your ego so you will be able to earn your living well, progress in the world well, compete with others and achieve your goals. For this purpose, it is really necessary that they train your ego in the "I" sense, for this sense of identity is necessary at a certain stage.

A spiritual teacher may say, "You must have a self-identity," and he might also say, "Lose yourself and be one with God." His statements appear to be contradictory, but they are not. One is losing the identity because you are sick, the other is losing your identity because you have chosen to do so. It is your wish, it is under your control. Whatever you give up consciously you can also take back consciously. If you know the switch, you can turn the light both on and off. But if the lights went on without your knowing about the switch, then you don't know how to turn the lights off or how to turn them on again. You are not in control. In mental illness, there is no control. One is a sickness while the other is transcendence.

Once you have established your ego, you are ready to go on a journey beyond the individual I to the cosmic I. This journey is taken in several stages. First are the people who are mentally and emotionally disturbed. They don't have an ego identity and so they need to learn how to establish one. Once this ego identity is established, they often become very successful in the world. The ego becomes like a drug. Just as certain drugs allow truck drivers to drive day and night, so the ego can make you work very hard on the material level. As you gain in the material world, however, you begin to lose in the subtle world of the spirit. When the spiritual lack becomes sufficiently acute, sufficiently painful, you are ready to transcend, ready to take a leap to another stage, from ego to non-ego, from ego to love.

At this point, you may go through a stage where you feel ineffective. Many people come to me and say, "What is happening to me? I used to be so effective in the world. Now suddenly I feel like I can't do anything." This is a necessary transitional stage which you may encounter before you enter the higher stage of love. You might not be able to produce as much as you did through ego, but that is fine because now you are trying to accomplish through love. Until your love becomes as strong as your ego, you may not get the same performance out of yourself.

One basic function of the guru, or spiritual teacher, is to guide you through the darkness of the tunnel as you move from having the ego as your center to having love as your center. You may go through a phase where you want to evade any further growth, and at this point, you may think that you want to go back to the known area of your ego. You know what happens there. It may be hell, but it is known, and you find comfort in that. The guru provides you with a setting and a surrounding, known as the ashram, or spiritual community. Through his company and through the company of loving brothers and sisters who take care of you when you go through this phase, you are able to rise to the level where you can draw your energy

28    from love. Without the guru, it is difficult to survive this phase. The strength of your past habits naturally draws you back into the ego and makes you feel comfortable there. Other people, even those who sincerely wish to help, cannot truly give you what you need at this stage, unless they themselves have grown beyond the ego. A psychiatrist, for example, would put you back into ego because that is the easy way to function—that is the way he knows. Only a guru who has himself grown into the realm of love can take you through the pain and suffering of ego so you may function with love energy.

As you attune yourself to this love energy, you become attuned to a universal, limitless source of energy. Drawing upon this love energy, you execute all actions with perfect harmony, perfect efficiency for the service of all humanity and for the love of all human beings. Once you have this energy, love exudes from your being as you work at peak performance. Love, happiness, enthusiasm, zest and joy flow from you as you hammer, as you type, as you walk. This is true energy. Having energy does not mean working with a long face; it does not mean getting your job done with tension, depression or anger. It means having love in action, performing each task as an act of service, without any ulterior motives, without any desire for benefit or recognition. If you can act from that state of consciousness, your work has become a form of love in action, an active worship of the God who dwells within you. Now your energy is drawn from love, rather than from ego. Now work can become play, an expression of joy from beginning to end. The man of love lives in such a state of consciousness, attuning himself to his inner love energy from moment to moment. He draws constantly on love as the highest source for all his daily activities, and in so doing, he establishes a life-line with the inexhaustible source of energy which is known as love.

# The Guru: A Vehicle
## for Transcending Attachment

**As you describe attachment, I can see that most of my relationships are attached relationships. Is there a possibility that these attachments can develop into love?**

There is always a possibility for attachment to blossom into love, but this is extremely difficult if both parties are in a relationship of attachment and if both are attached to each other. When both are absorbed in their own needs and expectations, it is difficult for either to see the needs of the other. Thus both become trapped in an on-going cycle of conflicting expectations and demands. Each feels threatened by the other, threatened that the other will not fulfill his own demands. Although they might appear to love one another, there is always an undercurrent of threat and fear. Somehow the cycle must be broken. If one partner in the relationship can learn to love freely and purely, he can then help the one who is attached to transcend his attachment. The liberated partner can then be a mirror for the one who is attached to help him grow above attachment. There must be one who has developed an objective awareness, who is established in the center, so that he can help the other to see himself and thus help him out of his problem. If both are attached, however, their condition is like that of the blind leading the blind.

**If I know I am attached, how can I grow past that attachment and learn to love freely and purely? What can I do to help this happen?**

You can only begin any journey from where you are. Most people are in the stage of attachment and not in love. If you want to grow into love, you must begin from where you are, you must begin with attachment. The secret is to attach yourself to the love of a person who has grown in love

30 on a high and pure level. Your attachment to such a person will gradually and steadily be transformed into pure love.

Love can only be learned through experience. Even when we are talking about love, love is still in the area of intellectual understanding. Love cannot be taught by lectures on love or through books on love. To grow into love, you must first experience being loved. I once heard a person recount the way she was taught about love. As a child, whenever she displayed anger, selfishness or jealousy, her parents gave her a book to read on love. Despite all her reading, she never learned to love—because she never was loved. Had she been loved, she would naturally have been loving.

Loving is not easy. If you are a novice in the art of love, you must be careful as to where you place your love. You will invariably be hurt if you start with the wrong person, in the wrong situation and for the wrong purpose. Others will take undue advantage of you and then you may quickly become disillusioned. In your disillusionment, you will naturally fear trying again. You will feel that the world is too selfish, that you don't want to be hurt, and so you will decide to treat the world as the world treats you. Instead of loving your neighbor as yourself, you will begin to hate your neighbor as you hate yourself.

Your nature is basically loving, but the energy which expresses itself through the heart has been blocked because of past experiences. That locked heart can only be opened through a relationship of pure love, by someone who has opened his own heart chakra. It can be opened only by someone who loves you with no conditions, no expectations, no strings attached—by someone who loves you as you are. Before you can fully open your heart and allow your love to flow, you must be able to trust fully.

There are few people whom you can trust so fully, few people who can love you purely and without conditions. In today's society, even those who are designated to provide guidance and assistance to others are themselves frequently starved for love. Teachers, therapists, doctors—

few of these people have grown beyond their own needs, conditions and expectations to the point where they can purely love the person who needs their help. Needless to say, there are doctors, therapists and others in the helping profession who do have the generosity, the purity and the capacity to truly help others learn about love. Many, however, lack this capacity because their relationship with students or patients is basically of a business nature, if not consciously, then subconsciously. The person coming for help knows this. He knows that if he doesn't provide the money or pay the fees, he will not receive help. As a result, he does not feel it is a pure relationship. His subconscious perception of the relationship as a business agreement blocks the flow of pure love and makes it difficult to develop the faith and trust which are needed to awaken love. Today's world has little love because there are so few people capable of imparting pure love through experience.

The guru, or spiritual teacher, is one who has grown to such a stage where he can be the center, the medium to awaken love. He has transcended the self-centered demands of the ego and senses. Because he has learned to love without conditions, he can provide you the experience of being loved and accepted as you are. As you begin to feel such total love, a unique thing happens. Suddenly you have the trust to love in return, suddenly you are able to open your heart and allow your trapped love to flow out. It is that very opening created when your love flows out which leaves the receptacle for you to receive love flowing in.

If you can find someone who loves you as you are, you can dare to love that person purely, without fears or inhibitions. If you find someone who accepts you as you are, you can learn to accept yourself. When you begin to accept yourself, you automatically begin to accept all others as well. This acceptance is true love—love without conditions or expectations. True love of another is total acceptance of that person. The guru facilitates your process of learning to love and accept others because he first loves and accepts you.

32     When you love someone, you are transformed without any conscious effort. When a boy loves a girl, he finds it easy to give up friends and habits she doesn't like. His love provides the impetus for change. He does not need to change consciously or with effort; his weaknesses simply begin to fall away. At one time, he may have lacked the initiative to hold a job, but now he can get up early in the morning to go to work. Because the money he receives through the job allows him to love the girl and give to her, holding a job becomes very easy for him. Even if he has difficulties on the job, he can bear with them because of the love he wants to fulfill.

A relationship of love can provide very spontaneous, effortless and sudden growth. If an ordinary relationship, based on attachment, can bring about such changes, higher love can work miracles. The love of the guru is a higher love. When you love a guru, his qualities begin to flow into you automatically and effortlessly. When your love for the guru becomes strong enough—when it becomes stronger than your demands or attachments—then those attachments are dissolved in his love. You become like the person you love. For this reason, you constantly intensify your love for the guru so that more and more attachments can be drowned in the ocean of his pure love. In this way the guru is able to absorb and eliminate all your problems.

The guru provides you with the possibility to love and to be loved. In this way, he becomes a gate, an entry into the kingdom of love. He becomes a catalytic agent that propels you into the higher states of consciousness through his love. The guru loves you purely. This love does everything else that is necessary. It takes up such a big space in your heart that there is no room for lower desires or self-destructive habits.

All that you experience is already within you. The guru does not give you anything which you don't already have; he simply awakens the pure love which lies within you, the pure love which is known as the inner guru. He removes

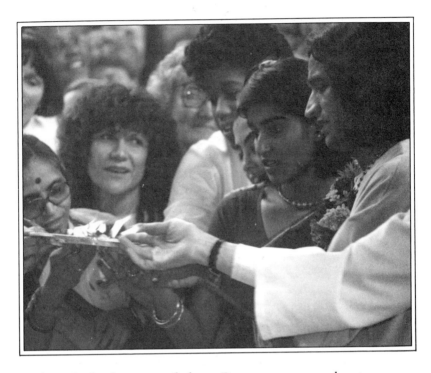

the veils that have curtailed you. Because you are so close to
yourself, you can't recognize the light of the inner guru
inside yourself. The external guru is one who mirrors your
inner guru so completely that you begin to truly see what
lies within you. The external guru is an empty valley; you
speak the inner secrets of your heart and they echo right
back to you. Because he himself is empty of conditions and
addictions, he becomes an external reflection of the self
that lies beneath your conditions and addictions—the self
that lies beyond your attachments. Thus the external guru
becomes the key to awakening the inner guru—the source
of love—inside you.

Love is not just giving; it is also receiving. Most people
find it difficult to accept anything without first giving
something in exchange for it. They don't want to take love
for free. The guru is willing to receive your love; he is
willing to accept your service and devotion because he
knows that when you give to him you become more able to

34      accept his love and guidance. Thus, even in receiving love, the guru is giving love to the disciple.

When you love the guru, you do yourself a favor. The guru does not need your service; he allows you to give service and devotion because he knows that it allows you to be more open and receptive to him, to more fully receive his guidance. Service and devotion are not the requirements of the guru; they are the needs of the disciple. Such service provides the opening, it establishes a contact of energy through which the guru flows into the disciple.

Loving the guru means loving yourself, because there is no difference between the guru and your true self, your inner self. The guru wants only one thing and that is your inner unfoldment, your inner happiness. His teachings and principles are a means to achieve this inner happiness. When you love him, these teachings become an automatic part of your life because this spontaneous blossoming of love manifests actively. If you love the guru, you love and practice what he teaches. Then the qualities of pure love—selfless service to all, dedication, contentment, joy and peace—become part of your life. When you love the guru, you are no longer fearful or tense. Instead you remain unruffled, tranquil and at ease in all you do. At the same time, you are able to work at peak performance because you are free of the non-acceptance and rejection which normally hinder your efforts. As a result, your blocks are removed and your capacity for peak performance is activated.

When you truly love the guru, that love can work miracles in your life. Because you are very open to him, his every word penetrates your consciousness so deeply that it has a capacity to totally transform your behavior and personality. In this love, there are no barriers of language or communication. This heart-to-heart communion bypasses the sentry of the mind which is normally clogged by preconceived ideas and prejudices. If you truly love the guru, you are open to the guru's guidance on both a verbal and a non-verbal level. In this total communion, the guru's energy flows to you constantly through the open channel of your love and trust for him. The guru's heart speaks to your heart, and you understand without the need for words, because you love him. This relationship can remove any obstacle; it can transform your life, it can open your love center. It is not the guru who is transforming you, however, it is your need to grow in love which has allowed you to be open to him. Both are necessary; the guru who is a vehicle to awaken your love and your own need to grow in love. The guru cannot give you more than you believe he is capable of giving. He simply provides the situation, the opportunity for you to awaken love. You are the one who must seize that opportunity and work with it, reverently and gratefully.

Those who lack this direct experience of love can practice the willful disciplines of yoga, gradually and with effort evolving to a stage where they can open their hearts. Those fortunate enough to experience the love of the guru, however, can be transformed quickly and effortlessly. This love is most readily available on the path of Shaktipat Kundalini Yoga, the path in which the guru transfers his actual, spiritual energy to the ready disciple. With this transferral, the disciple experiences a spontaneous and effortless awakening of love for the guru. The energy of Shakti is love energy. It automatically opens your heart and transforms your life by awakening you into pure love.

Love is the only ingredient that can so totally transform you, yet without the guru, this love is hard to experience. For this reason, it is very difficult to grow fully into your higher nature of love without the love and guidance of a guru.

**You talk about attachment and you talk about love for the guru. Isn't that just another form of attachment?**

Love for anyone inevitably begins with attachment. Even when you love the right person with a higher motive,

36  your love is still an attached love, because attachment is what you know. If your attachment is to a person who is himself attached and who does not know how to gradually wean you from him, you become further attached. You will both be attached, and it will be difficult for either to grow beyond attachment. But if you first become attached to one who has transcended attachment, to one who has opened his heart chakra, then your attachment can gradually develop into pure, non-attached love.

The guru loves you in the highest manner because he loves you in an objective and compassionate way. He has learned to look at the world, to look at himself, in an objective way and so he can also look at you with objectivity. This objectivity is not indifference, it is a loving awareness, a compassionate non-attachment. Because he is not attached to you, the guru can understand your problems and your attachments without becoming emotionally upset or disillusioned by your weaknesses. Because he expects nothing from you, he can truly help you.

In the initial stages you will be attached to the guru, but this attachment will eventually lead you beyond all attachment. For that reason, it is an attachment of the highest nature. When you become sufficiently attached to the guru, when you become totally absorbed in him, you become one with him. Your inner guru is then fully activated and you recognize that the guru whom you love so deeply is within you. Then all attachment dissolves and you enter into the realm of pure and non-attached love. The guru is like a train. When you travel by train you are attached to and dependent upon the train until you reach your destination. Once you have reached your goal, however, you don't cling to the train. So it is with attachment to the guru. Once your inner guru has become fully awakened, you experience the guidance and love of the guru from within. Now there is no attachment, there is only pure and total love between the guru and the disciple.

**Why must this process happen through a guru? I love my wife and she is a good person. Can't the same thing happen through my loving her? Can't it happen through love for my child or through love of God?**

If your love for anyone is strong enough, that love can activate your inner guru. If you love your wife in the highest manner, she can activate your inner guru. If you love your child in the highest manner, your inner guru can be awakened. But can you love them in the highest manner? It will be difficult because you are attached to them and they are attached to you. Neither will find it easy to break the habit patterns of conditions and expectations to become truly loving. Your demands and expectations of each other will invariably curtail perfect love. For this reason you need a guru, one who is himself non-attached, who can accept your attachment without becoming attached to you.

You may also awaken your inner guru by holding God in your heart, but this is a difficult path for most people. God is abstract—you can't see him, and so it is difficult to truly experience his love for a sustained period of time. Since you do not really know God, it is difficult to focus upon him. It is much easier to go through his agent—through someone who can provide direct guidance and a concrete example to you. The guru is such a person. When Master Christ said, "The man who has seen me has seen the Father . . . I am in the Father and the Father is in me." (John 14: 8-9), he was speaking as a perfect guru—a pure channel for the love of God. God is already within you, but he can most easily be uncovered, he can most easily be known, by experiencing the pure love and guidance of an external guru.

## 38   The Art of Daily Loving

**Gurudev, I never seem to receive much love from others and yet I know I need love. Can you tell me how I can draw more of the love I need, how I can receive more love from others?**

Your problem comes from placing your emphasis in the wrong place, but this is natural. Most people do this. Let me explain.

Man always wants to be loved, he wants to be understood. This desire is a selfish one, one which only takes him further from the love he craves. He becomes so engrossed in his own needs that he fails to see the needs of anyone else. Thus, his craving for love is self-defeating because it makes him less and less capable of relating to anyone. He cuts off all communication channels with others because he is always looking at them as potential objects for his fulfillment. He turns the whole world into an object for satisfaction. In so doing, he feels even more lonely, fearful, tense, and defensive—all in the name of wanting love.

There is only one way to receive love—and that is by giving love. When you give love freely, and without expectation of return, then you are truly able to receive love. Most people measure the love they give carefully and watch closely to see if it is returned with equal measure. There is no way to measure love, for love given with a desired return is not love. It is a contract. If you want love badly, then give love totally, with no thought of receiving anything. Then love will come to you.

When you are concerned about others, when you want to help others, you will never feel bad yourself. This is the secret. People who get depressed are very selfish people. They can only see their problems and pay no attention to the needs of those around them. Those who really care for others can never afford depressions. When a bad mood comes, they immediately come out of it because they are not concerned with their own desires and disappointments.

Their love for others keeps them too busy to worry about themselves. This is why true love is the greatest source of joy, not so much to the receiver, but to the giver of love.

When you give love, you are providing security to others. You are caring for them, providing comfort and ease to them. As a result, you do not expect negative vibrations. You have no reason to fear the other, because you have made him so secure that he has no reason to threaten you. When you expect and demand something from the other, the other becomes a threat. And, as a result, you expect negative vibrations and you will be defensive and fearful. Thus, providing security brings you security and demanding security robs you of security.

Most people believe that love comes from someone outside themselves. This is a great fallacy, a fallacy responsible for much pain and suffering in the world. No one can give you what you don't already have. You could be the most loved person on this earth, but if you don't love yourself, you will be miserable. There is only one way to love yourself, and that is to provide love to others. So when I say, "Love yourself," don't misunderstand. Always know that loving yourself means providing love to others.

Instead of artificially trying to draw love from others, first learn to accept yourself. Anyone can create the false feeling of acceptance and belonging by commanding it from some outside source, but only the person of true depth and maturity can find acceptance within. Learn to accept yourself and everyone else will accept you as well. Learn to accept yourself and you will naturally accept all others. Then only can you experience true love—love which is free from fear, dependence and attachment. This love can begin by accepting both yourself and others at the same time. Eventually, you will have to put more accent on loving others. Then your love will gradually begin to come back to you. Do not give love with the intention that it will come back to you however. Love given with expectation of return is not pure love. As soon as you expect a certain

40     return, you become attached to the results of your love. You must establish yourself in true love by removing any expectations that you will receive anything from giving love. This is a very key point.

A student once asked me the question, "Guruji, you are surrounded by so many disciples who love you so much. How can you take all the love you receive from people? Most people simply couldn't contain that much love." I can only receive love because I can give it—that's the secret. If love was constantly coming to me and I didn't give it to others, it would feed my ego and take away my capacity to love. Love cannot be kept. It cannot be made stagnant, because love is energy. Energy must constantly move. It expands as it is given, as it is distributed and shared. When people love me, I don't try to hold onto their love and make it mine. I receive it only to expand it and to immediately share it with many others who are thirsty for love.

**Gurudev, I work with a lot of people, sometimes under pressure, and often personality conflicts arise. This happens also with my family. What is the best way to resolve these conflicts?**

You have a beautiful built-in system for finding out what your problems are. Simply find out who you dislike and then carefully examine why you dislike him. If you are perceptive, you will quickly discover that this person has something you want or that he reminds you of some aspect of yourself which you dislike in yourself. When you examine the person you dislike, you will know what you want to be. This principle applies to jealousy and competition as well. You can only be jealous of someone who represents what you want to be. If you lack the capacity to fulfill your own expectations of yourself, you fill the void by hating or becoming jealous of the person who is successful in being what you want to be. You initially created the desire to be other than what you are. Now, because you can't have what you desire, you compensate for your own lack by hating someone else. Then you think you've solved the problem.

Whenever you compare yourself with anyone, you create a psychological void. The easiest way to fill that void is by hating the person you've selected as an object for your comparison. When you compete, the same process occurs. In order to find a partner for your competition, you choose someone whom you feel is already better than you. Then you compete to prove to yourself that you are better than him. You can never win in this game because at the outset you have already accepted the fact that he is better. Now all your efforts are directed at destroying a concept which you yourself have created.

Why should you compare yourself with anyone? Only God is perfect, everyone else is imperfect. Why disturb yourself worrying if someone is more efficient, more advanced or less imperfect than you in a given area? That will not help you grow. Just simply be what you are. Enter into a relationship of love with one who is awakened and established in his love center, with one who is non-attached and selfless in his service. That person doesn't necessarily have to be called a guru. He doesn't have to come from India, or be a yogi or another Jesus. A guru is one who has himself awakened his love center—whether he is known as a guru or not makes no difference. If you are associated with such a person, you are associated with a guru.

The lower your self-image, the more you will dislike others and compete with others. The stronger you become, the less will be your need to compete or compare. Could you imagine an elephant wanting to fight with ants? He can crush millions of ants with one stamp of his foot, so why should he even bother to fight? Become a spiritual elephant, so strong in your love and self-acceptance that you never need to prove your worth at the expense of anyone.

When you encounter someone you would ordinarily dislike, find out why you dislike that person and then learn to love him. In reality, you can never hate anyone unless

42     you also love that person. Since your love is attached, however, since it is interwoven in your own insecurities and demands, it becomes hate. When you experience hate for someone, know that you have come into possession of a valuable key. That key can do two things: it can lock the door of your heart or it can open it. The same energy, the same hate, that locks your heart can be transformed into equally powerful love to open your closed door. You must face your hate, however, if you want to go beyond it. If you say, "I don't want to look at my hate, I want to stay away from it," then you will never unlock your love. If the key hates the lock, it will never open the door. First face your hate, then dissolve it through understanding.

Your dislike for another person invariably stems from your own dislike of yourself. Whenever you dislike some part of yourself, you will dislike those who have the same qualities as well as those who are what you want to be. In the same manner, another person's dislike of you is the result of their own self-rejection. For this reason, never accept anyone's dislike of you. Instead, have compassion for their own dislike of themselves.

When you hate someone, you enter into an imaginary exchange of anger with that person. Actually you create an entity and then you enter into a conversation with that entity. You put words in his mouth and then you argue with him. Before you transfer your anger onto him, you prepare the facts to suit your interpretation of the situation. Because you never actually deal with the other person about the incident which caused the anger, however, you never have a chance to resolve it. Now you are stuck with all the imaginary arguments that you have created. When you imagine yourself inflicting pain and suffering onto him through your words, you release a number of chemical poisons in your own body, thereby becoming the victim of your own imagination, your own anger. After all your imaginary confrontations, you rarely dare to share your feelings with others because you are not sure you will say it right and that it will be heard correctly, yet you continue to suffer the consequences of your own inner negativity.

Knowing this, stop your inner imaginary fights and begin to love those who dislike you. Everyone needs love. If you can truly love, even the most negative person will accept your love. There is no human being alive who cannot respond to love in some form. You can never love too much, but you can love too much in your own way, in a way that the other may not understand. When you want to love another, you must love him on his level, in a way that he can accept and understand. Then he won't feel threatened by your love.

When you find it difficult to communicate with someone, begin to dwell on that person's beautiful qualities. Each day spend time recalling the good qualities of that person. By and by your very gestures, the very words you speak to him and the way you look at him will begin to change. He will instinctively feel your love, without your telling him that you love him. Then he will begin to change. In the same way, if you speak constant words of love to a person and yet entertain negative thoughts about him, he will hear the true story. He will not need to be a psychologist to read your hidden language.

If your love is superficial, if it masks negative thoughts, the other will feel your true dislike. For this reason, it is essential to think only positive thoughts about others. Such positive thinking is the major secret of good relations with others.

**I really want to learn to be more loving in a very concrete way in my daily life. Can you give me some specific suggestions?**

That's a beautiful question. Do you remember when we talked about what love is not? You do not need to know what love is in order to practice love. You need only to drop that which is not love from your life. Drop as many nega-

44   tive qualities as you can. Then you will be gradually transformed into love. You know that hatred is not love, that
jealousy is not love, that violence is not love. In that case,
begin to practice non-violence; remove the hatred, jealousy
and competition from your life. Learn to dissolve your
personal desires and interests. To whatever extent you
remove selfishness, to that extent you will be a loving
person. Consciously undertake activities that are intended
to serve God, to serve humanity, to serve your guru and all
others. You will become a loving person.

Eric Fromm describes love as an art. There are things
you must do to become proficient at any art, and love is no
exception. According to Fromm, any aspiring artist must
begin by disciplining himself, by practicing concentration
and patience. Fromm is correct. Certain desciplines are most
necessary to the person who would master the art of love.

Love requires continuous practice and the best place to
begin practicing is with yourself. When you acquire the art
of loving yourself, you naturally love others as well. Many
people beat themselves psychologically day and night. They
use the weapons of tension, anxiety, guilt and fear. Such
self-hate does not allow you to love others. If you are in
love with yourself, you hate no one. You are neither tense
nor fearful. Relaxation is a by-product of self-love. If you
are relaxed you are loving. Therefore, if you find it difficult
to love, work on becoming relaxed. Learn to give love rather than expect it and you will be relaxed. Remain in a non-
expectant state of consciousness and you will be relaxed.

The disciplines of yoga are designed to help you become relaxed—to help you love yourself. Practiced with
perseverance and concentration, they will gradually lead
you from suffering and pain on each level of your being—
physical, mental, emotional and spiritual. Because they are
designed to release deep-set tensions, they also remove the
corresponding patterns of mental and emotional disturbance, fear and self-rejection which always accompany tension. Through a balanced program of hatha yoga

exercises, breathing techniques, meditation, relaxation, proper diet, karma yoga (the yoga of non-attached action) and bhakti yoga (the yoga of love and devotion), along with the mental and moral observances known as Yama and Niyama, you will soon experience new levels of energy, and with it, increased satisfaction, peace and ease.

As you apply all the various techniques of yoga to your life, you must at the same time remain in the relaxed state of consciousness which is called contentment. Being content does not mean being lazy or lethargic, it means accepting yourself as you are. When contentment is the undercurrent behind all activity, it releases a greater amount of energy to deal with any given situation more effectively than ever before. This contentment is the experience of loving yourself—your higher self. As you experience it to greater and greater degrees, you are ready to begin loving others in a true sense.

As you progress in your mastery of love, you will need to change your habitual attitudes and ways of viewing the world. No longer can you afford to reject anyone based on your own value system or concepts of how they should be. No longer can you afford to entertain negative thoughts about others. Instead live creatively and positively, developing new habits and new experiences. Learn to drop your expectations and desires of others. When you have no desires, you have no fears. Then you have room for love to enter. If you would learn to love, you must learn to accept that external conditions always change. There is no way you can ever establish ideal external conditions and expect those conditions to stay the same forever. To have a relationship with someone and hope it always remains a certain way is sheer foolishness. If you are not the same from one minute to the next, how can you expect someone else to be? When you fully understand the law of change and accept it as an integral part of your life, when you live expecting nothing from anyone, then you are truly adjusting to everyone at all times. You are truly loving everyone at all times.

46    Loving is complete flexibility. It is adjusting, adapting and accepting anything and everything that happens to you and around you at any given time. This is what yogis call surrender. This is living the expression, "Thy will be done, not mine." To be loving is to be surrendered, to live in attunement with the Divine will. Thus the man who has awakened his heart chakra, the man who has learned to love purely, lives in total attunement with the Divine. That attunement is love in the highest sense.

Discover how it feels to love someone. Discover the transforming effect upon your own life through working for others. Discover the ecstasy and newness of giving freely rather than desiring to receive. Learn to enjoy giving. Once you learn to do so, giving is even more of a joy than receiving. Seeing the ecstasy and the joy of the other will naturally provide an opening in your heart. Seeing the joy others receive through your love will open up a new dimension in your life, and you will discover that life has much more to give than you ever dreamed possible.

Start with doing small favors with no expectation of reward. You will find such fulfillment that you will naturally want to do more and more favors. Soon your sincere desire will be to love, rather than to be loved. Now the love you give will be reflected back to you, and you will feel secure in the certainty that you are loved.

What a beautiful thing it is to fall in love with the whole world, to find that there is nothing outside your love. When you love like this, you bring God through your love. Then God is working through you, because to whatever extent you experience love, to that extent you are in touch with God within you. Then your limited love becomes a vehicle to carry you to the highest, purest love. Then your love becomes God fully manifest, through you, through each and every action that you perform.

# Postscript

"Blessed are the meek, for they shall inherit the earth." The meek person is the humble, honest, compassionate and loving person. The power-hungry mind cannot be loving. The prestige-seeking mind cannot be honest. The love-seeking mind cannot be loving, honest or at peace. Love is found by giving and not by seeking. Giving is receiving, but seeking is losing. Seeking begins from the other, but love begins from you, for you are the center of the universe. When you ask love of others you lose your center, you lose your freedom, you lose the bliss of your true nature. You become addicted to external objects. When sought from outside, love becomes hate and violence. Look within for the true source of love. Internally you will become free—non-expectant, non-dependent and free from demands for love. Then your love will blossom.

True seeking is providing—providing love to others. Open the gate of your love to give. Let your heart become a great generator of love and then love will come back to you. Only when you give love will you ever receive love, for love begins from you. Give totally. Totally detach yourself from all expectations of the world outside. God within will provide all. You will be the king of kings, not a destitute beggar. Stop all asking and you will inherit the kingdom of heaven. Give up all external things and the God within you, the love within you, will come alive. Then you will become one with God.

# Guru and Disciple:
## A Relationship of Love

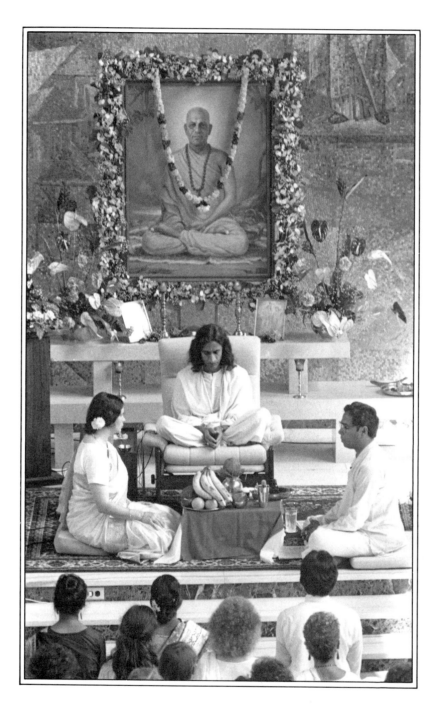

# The Guru: A Definition

*A guru is one who teaches what he has realized directly.*

No verbal communication is necessary once you love. No distance exists between people once you love. All relationships become simple when love is present. It makes no difference how this love develops. It can grow through a friend, a husband, or a wife, but there must be a single person to whom you can give your love fully, fearlessly. You must know that your love will not be misused, for fear will keep you from loving. If it will keep you from loving, it will also keep you from being loved. To find a person in whom you can completely, wholeheartedly place your love without the fear of it being abused is most difficult. There are few people who can accept your love and trust without selfish motivation. The guru (spiritual teacher) is one who has this capacity. He facilitates your ability to love by creating a situation in which your love and trust can grow.

The guru has become what you aspire to be. He has gone through many difficulties, he has traveled the intricate paths of growth, he has encountered life's problems. He says, "My son, if you want to walk with me, just follow me." To follow him is to follow his life. For the guru is not his body, the guru is what he has digested in his life. He is not merely a professor or a teacher. A teacher can be an intellectual. He can study and he can teach you, but he may never have experienced what he teaches. The guru is one who has experienced what he teaches and who teaches what he has realized directly. His guidance helps you eliminate mistakes and grow quickly on the spiritual path.

The guru is a vehicle for your spiritual growth, for you to work out your problems and give up your ego. He becomes a mirror for you. When you stand in front of him, he reflects whatever you are. But as you move away, he does not hold on to that reflection. When someone else comes to him, they will see only their own image and not the images

52    of others. The guru does not hold any concepts or beliefs about you. He is continuously open to any human being in any situation.

The guru is a gate through which you pass. He provides an outlet for you; he is a catalytic agent; he stirs that which is already within you. The search for a guru leads you within. It is said, "When the disciple is ready, the guru appears." That is the same as saying, "Necessity is the mother of invention." "Ask and ye shall receive. Knock and it shall be opened to you." When you are ready, your inner guru will be awakened and you will be able to recognize the right external guru for you.

The real guru is the God that resides in the temple of your body. He is the guru of all gurus. External gurus are merely representatives of that guru within. An external guru will be useless to you if your inner guru has not been awakened to some small degree. But you need an external guru to fully activate your inner guru.

When your inner guru is activated, you can follow any discipline without flaw; you can remain calm in the midst of disturbance; you can remain centered in the midst of problems; you can remain balanced in the midst of both success and failure. When you have such balance and harmony, your inner guru has awakened fully. Until then you must seek the guidance of an external guru if you are to grow in the quickest manner.

### Guru—a Word and a Role

A true guru does not consider himself to be a guru. In order to communicate with you, however, he uses the word "guru" because that word breaks through your usual mental associations. If he uses the word "friend", you will think of your associations with friends—how they treated you and what their friendship meant to you. If he calls himself a teacher, you will very likely recall your student days and think of a teacher in a classroom. That would create a misconception. It would be little better for him to call himself a guide, because there are many guides who take you through many different subjects. When you go on a trip, there are guides who take you sightseeing through museums. Each of these words is a symbol which represents certain things according to your past experiences. Each conveys a concept which is limited for you by your value system, habits, and preconceived ideas.

The word "guru" is also a symbol—a symbol which is connected to very special meanings and associations in the Eastern world. It communicates a certain idea which is not clearly communicated by words such as "teacher", "guide", or "friend". And so we use the word "guru" as a symbol—a symbol of a relationship which is of the highest nature. You could call the guru your friend, brother, father, or fellow traveler on the path of life. It makes no difference what you call it, so long as the relationship is capable of awakening the divine force within you, so long as it fulfills the function of the guru-disciple relationship. Such a relationship encompasses all other relationships. It fills the role of mother, father, friend, teacher, and guide.

## The Search for a Guru

*Seeking is defining. You must know what you are seeking when you are seeking.*

In the search for love, in the search for freedom, man fell into bondage. The need for exciting things, newer things, better things, is the need for love. When man couldn't get true love, he filled that gap with various substitutes and ended up with many self-destructive desires. Then man became the victim of these desires, despite the fact that he was searching only for love. He became bound to people, bound to things, attached to people, attached to things, but in this attachment he did not find the true love he was seeking.

54    There are three kinds of people: people who are asleep, people who are searching, and people who are awake. The majority belong to the first class, some belong to the second class, and to the third class, the awake, few truly belong.

The man who is in the state of sleep and ignorance appears to be happy; he appears to be content with his dream world. But this appearance of happiness and contentment is false. The man asleep acts out his stereotyped, everyday routine and hopes a miracle will change his life. This type of man is represented by the first chakra, the Muladhara Chakra. He sees little significance to his life. He sees no way out, nor does he want to put forth any effort to get out. He is lazy—he is asleep.

The second type of man has suffered the blows of destiny. He has gone through the problems of life, he has encountered the difficulties of life, he has come up against the walls of life, and he questions, "Is this all that life is about?" Then he begins to awaken; he begins to search. He tries to find a person who can enhance that search that is beginning to dawn faintly in his consciousness.

Yet, man does not know exactly what he is looking for, so in his search he tries many things. The man who is just beginning to search will first look through material objects. He thinks that if he has more money he will be able to buy happiness. He purchases many things: power, recognition, sex—all sorts of satisfaction.

The second chakra represents this man who is in search of lust fulfillment. He goes everywhere trying to find the object of his desire, trying all sorts of material methods to satisfy his sensual wants. But after acquiring some degree of satisfaction he finds that it is not enough. Then he searches for power. He enters the realm of the third chakra, which represents the power principle. He tries to find inner satisfaction through the manipulation of power in his job, his marriage, his friends, and his wealth.

The man who has begun to awaken realizes the futility and uselessness of that search for power and sensual gratification. He begins to look for the higher meaning of life. He flies up to the fourth chakra, the heart chakra, and catches a glimpse of the divine joy which radiates through the heart. But despite his sincerity he has not yet found enough guidance and inspiration to be consistent in his search. As a result his energy may drop and he again is drawn by gravity to the lower chakras which represent the misuse and loss of energy. He begins to feel insecure in his search for security, he looks for a way to hide from his higher nature. He takes shelter in sensual gratification and a superficial search for God. He uses sex, he watches television, he reads religious books, he attends spiritual lectures, he eats a vegetarian diet. He finds many, many different devices in which to hide, in which to feel secure. But soon he becomes disappointed in these devices. He looks around at others and realizes that nothing worthwhile is happening in their lives. He sees that their greater successes only bring greater insecurities. Then his eyes begin to open and the search for the guru begins.

## True Search and False Search

During the early stage of this search, in the name of searching for a path and a guru, man tries a variety of paths, techniques, gurus and methods in the hope of finding the right path, the right guru. But since he is searching for knowledge in the usual manner, he becomes a collector of information, growth techniques, and methods. He often carries the false notion, so common to a novice aspirant, that he believes in the universality of paths. Under this delusion he goes from one path to another, one guru to another, one technique to another, hoping to find the right one. But he does not have enough patience or perseverance to practice any one path with faith for a sustained period in order to test its validity. Such a spiritual search is common in the West where memory, or a collection of borrowed words and techniques, is confused with wisdom, direct

56     illumination, and experience.

If man continues to merely replace his collections of money, power, possessions, and sense objects with a collection of spiritual books and spiritual lectures—if he goes guru hopping and shopping—he again begins the same cycle of attachments and hide-outs. The only difference is that now it is all transferred to the spiritual ego, to spiritual pride and collection, to spiritual competition. He has replaced one kind of materialism with another. He goes from one type of collection to another and thinks of himself as a spiritual seeker, but he is not.

There is a time for sincerely seeking a path, but there is also a time to settle and practice one. This is the secret that the average seeker does not understand. He keeps running all his life, thinking he is so smart. He goes to all the spiritual lectures, he reads all the spiritual books, but he practices nothing. Follow one path. Do this, not because other paths are wrong, but because it is necessary that you follow one path in order to truly realize that there is truth in all other paths. Respect everyone, but do not distract yourself in the name of respect and freedom. In the name of freedom you follow one path, then you follow another path, you study this technique and you study another technique, and you get distracted. The mind has to be applied in one direction.

It is like a businessman who starts a clothing business and then says, "I believe in free enterprise. I want to start in the stock market." Then he immediately changes his mind again and starts a car business. He will lose money everywhere. He has to establish himself in one business and go deep enough, lose money in the earlier stage, and then start making money. That is true in any search, whether it is a search for money, name, fame, or spiritual growth. You have to hold yourself to one path and follow it thoroughly, respecting others, having love and understanding for all paths, but practicing one. Take the example of the man who digs fifty holes two feet deep in search of water. He cannot hope to be successful by digging so many shallow holes. To do that he must dig one hole one hundred feet deep. Then he has a chance to find water. You must follow one path and dig one hole deep enough to get the water of spiritual growth. Then you will truly recognize the unity of all men.

Practice one path thoroughly until you get results. Someone once asked me, "What is the best meditation technique?" I said, "There is no one technique that is better than any other; all techniques are merely techniques. They gain their strength and usefulness from the practitioner. The technique which is practiced with dedication, persistence, and perseverance is the best technique." So also the path you follow with total dedication is the best path for you.

How do you recognize the right path, the right guru? As long as a guru is practicing and growing and is not distracted, he can be a guide for you. If someone says, "I only want the perfect master. I don't want anything else.", he will have a difficult search. How are you going to know who is a perfect master? You will never know. It takes a thief to catch a thief. You will have to be a perfect master to recognize one. Don't worry about recognizing a perfect master. A guru who can inspire you, who always follows the highest path, who is one-pointed in his search, who stands for the highest in everyone, who never denounces anyone, who is motivated by the divine, such a guru will always help. He doesn't have to be an enlightened master. If you grow beyond him you can then find a more advanced guru.

Just as a tree can be judged by its fruit, so a guru can be known by looking at his disciples. You meet the children and you know the parents. The one whose company you keep is the one you become like. Find the right company, let yourself trust fully, and as you grow you will know whether he is the right guru or not. But without trusting, without growing in his teachings, you will never know if he is the right guru for you. The flowers are always fragrant, but you must come close to smell their sweet scent. The fragrance of a guru comes through his teachings, through

58    your open heart. He continually spreads his scent of love, but you must be open to receive it.

## The Role of the Guru

*As the guru acts, so he teaches.*

Spiritual experiences are valuable only under instruction. Many people have spiritual experiences without guidance and instruction, but such experiences can become detrimental to your growth if they are misused or misinterpreted. The value of spiritual experiences is in what you receive from them, how you use them. No matter what good experiences you have, if you don't recognize them, they are useless to you. If you find a diamond, but don't recognize it as a diamond, then to you it is a piece of glass. It is of no value to you and you will throw it away. You must have a physical guru if you are to recognize the value of your experiences. The role of the guru is to guide you through these experiences so that you may grow beyond them. That is why the guru is necessary.

There is no way you can make it on the higher path without a guru, because this path is full of intricacies. A process of growth that would take you six months, six years, or sometimes a whole lifetime can be accomplished with his one look. You come to him and you ask him questions. He may give you a simple answer. You may not even suspect that he has helped, but he may have erased many problems in your heart. Just his love can do it. Follow his guidance and be happy with it. There are many difficulties which can come on this path. If you are to save your time and energy, if you are to grow quickly, you must follow the guidance of a guru implicitly.

### The Purpose of a Guru

The average spiritual seeker believes many foolish notions about things that he has read from books. This is a great weakness. He reads that you don't need a guru or that the guru is within you, that God is within. He rejoices in those words while his life continues to stink. His life has no zest, no purity, no joy, no growth. Still he holds onto that belief and says, "God is within me." It is ridiculous. "God is within me" is a wonderful philosophy and it is true, but you have to have a vantage point to realize God within you. The guru becomes this vantage point, a gate to higher growth. If you are studying piano, what is the value of your piano teacher? You will learn to play the piano if you keep at it for many years. You will eventually reach a certain standard, but the purpose of your teacher is to bring you to that same level within a short time. The purpose of the guru is to shorten the suffering, to shorten the fear, to protect the disciple.

The guru shows you your problem spots, he shows you where the dead ends are. He shows you how to grow at a higher speed with fewer problems. God has given you both energy and the choice of how to handle it. You have an absolute choice, but you haven't exercised that choice for so long that you don't know how to use your energy. This is called ignorance. We have the freedom of choice, yet we do not exercise it. We have used certain methods and practices so habitually in the past that we have forgotten how to use our energy in a higher way. This is why it is necessary to have a guru—an awakened person—who has already used higher methods, who knows your problems and your hurdles, who can remove them one after another.

The guru's responsibility is to make you aware, to awaken love within you. But it is not the guru who is doing it. All he does is provide you with the love. The love itself does everything. Psychologically the love of a guru gives you the greatest strength to grow, to go through the most difficult problems.

The guru's love is not an emotional love, an ego-centered love. An emotional love, because it is sensual, excites you and depresses you since excitement and depression cannot be separated. But the guru's love is beyond both excitement and depression, because it is an unconditional love. All the guru wants is the disciple's growth.

The guru projects himself, his behavior, his actions and his lifestyle in such a way that it constantly provides the disciple with the possibility of recognizing the love and faith that lie dormant within him. If he can do that he doesn't need to teach anything. That faith and love will automatically do the teaching. What can be taught with the tongue will not stand the test of time, it will be worn out, but what can be taught with deep love will never be forgotten.

You start from the outside with the external guru, but you don't stay outside. By and by the guru's guidance becomes internalized, it becomes your experience. Your inner guidance becomes active because of your direct experience. Now the external guidance becomes an experience, an inspiration, an inner guidance.

Though you may feel the presence of your inner guru, you can feel his guidance only when you are functioning from your heart. When your inner guru goes to the head and you become intellectual you begin to have doubts. This is when you need an external guru. Your internal guru is always present, but his guidance is available only when you function through your heart. As long as your inner guru fluctuates from your heart to your head you will need the guidance of an external guru. When you begin to respond fully with your heart your inner guru will remain awakened all the time. Then the external guru has fulfilled his purpose. Externally he is no longer necessary because he now resides within you.

### Awakening the Inner Guru

Awakening, not teaching, is the key. Once you are awakened, all teachings flow from within through the inner guru. To be awakened is to have the inner guru awakened. The external guru is needed to awaken the inner guru. You must learn how to get to the source which becomes the guru for you. That true guru is the highest consciousness that dwells within you—the guru of all gurus. The external guru functions as a vehicle to activate and awaken this inner guru. For most people the darkness is so powerful that they cannot awaken their inner guru. Before you can see the light within, you must search for the light outside. When you recognize the light in someone else you know where to go. Recognizing that light in someone else is also your inner awakening. Then you can spot your external guru. You are drawn to an external guru who, in turn, helps to draw out your internal guru.

In the early stages your inner guru is awakened only momentarily. In this awakened state you recognize your external guru, you feel an attraction for him, and you approach him to become his disciple. You do not, however, stay in this awakened state.

Your partially awakened inner guru guides you to the external guru who then further awakens your internal guru. You will not go in search of a guru unless your inner guru is awakened to some degree for a short period of time. At that time you see the need to grow. You see the beauty in the guru who can inspire you, who can guide you on the higher path.

The very fact that you are searching for a guru, that you can see beauty and love in others, means you are thirsty for growth. It means that your inner guru has begun to awaken. But for that small light passing through you to grow larger, you need an external guru through whom the light is shining fully. Your partially awakened inner guru will not be awake all the time. You need an external guru who can uncover your inner guru through his blessings, his love, his actions and his guidance. By establishing contact with such a guru, by loving him and surrendering to him, your inner guru will be fully uncovered until his light is shining fully.

62     The first guru is within you. But if you open your heart to someone whom you respect and love, who has already reached the heights to which you aspire, then you are strengthening and helping yourself. The process varies, but the end result is one and the same—either you awaken the guru within by being totally aware of yourself or you awaken him through the help of a person who is totally aware.

To awaken that inner guru through an external guru, your attitude toward the external guru becomes most significant. Everything you feel toward that external guru is going to affect your progress. Your respect for him is your respect for the guru within. Your surrender to the external guru is surrender to the guru within. The way you love your external guru is the way you are beginning to love yourself.

The awakening of the inner guru begins by following the disciplines given by the external guru. You have to obey the external guidance of a guru before you can truly experience the guidance of your inner guru. The inner guru is always aware, but to recognize him you need the confirmation and support of the external guru.

Only when your inner guru is awakened to some degree will you begin to love your external guru. Then by loving your external guru you will begin to love your internal guru with more depth and devotion. Then again your external guru will begin to appeal to you. He will begin to flow into you and awaken your true guru within at deeper and deeper levels. You can then attune yourself more fully to the energy of the external guru. This guru becomes a continuous inspiration, even when you leave him physically. If you love him you can command his presence by remembering his way of living, thinking, and acting. It is this love which establishes the energy link between the disciple and the guru, the inner connection which hastens and supports the disciple's growth.

This link can be established with anyone. If you can love your wife thoroughly, your inner guru will be awakened; if you love your child in the highest manner, your inner guru will be awakened. It is not the object of love, but how you love that is important to your growth. Most relationships of this nature cannot facilitate your higher growth because you are attached to the other person and they are attached to you. That attachment keeps you from love, because attachments always curtail true love. An attached love is a conditional love. That is why you have to have a guru who is non-attached, who can love you without being attached to you on an ego level. If he is attached to you he won't be able to see any of your problems, nor will he be able to help you. An awakened person, who has grown beyond attachment, who has used the higher methods, who knows where your problems are, where your hurdles are, can remove them one after the other.

But first you must surrender to that awakened person, to the guru. If you can surrender to a stone statue, that statue can become a guru to you. The question is: where can you surrender? Can you surrender to a God you cannot see? For most people that is difficult. But it is easier to surrender to a living person whose life commands your love and trust. Such a person is the guru.

A guru cannot give you more than you think he is capable of giving. Even if he is God Himself, he is totally helpless if you don't think he can do anything for you. It is you who is giving energy to God to become God. God is first within you, the guru is first within you. Unless you surrender yourself to him, unless you trust him, trust yourself, trust the guru within you, you will never truly grow. It is not the guru, but your surrender to him, your faith and trust in him, which are the primary ingredients for your growth.

## Love and Dependence

The love between a guru and a disciple is the highest love. There is nothing on earth that can be compared with that love. It is the highest because it takes you to the

64 highest level of consciousness.

Once you have love for the guru, he can do anything for you. Don't worry about your attachment or your non-attachment to him. If the love transforms you, if it changes you, you can call it attachment and it makes no difference. Attachment to the right person, performed with awareness, lifts you out of attachment. The guru can help you because he is not attached to you. In the earlier stages do not try to distinguish between love and attachment. Just love your guru as much as you can, surrender to him as much as you can. As long as the guru remains non-attached he can transform your attachment into pure love.

You can become non-attached only by first being attached. You can jump into the ocean only if you are on the ground. You can become relaxed only if you are tense. You can become happy only if you are upset. You must experience attachment and understand it. Then only can you give it up. Attachment is good as a stage of growth, because if you love your guru or you are attached to your guru, you will become attached to what he is, to what he teaches. He teaches good things. If you love him and want to maintain that attachment, you will need to do the things which he teaches. If you keep doing these things, you will eventually attain freedom. The guru represents the higher way of life. If you become attached to him, you become attached to this higher way of life. Then the guru helps you become established in the higher love.

So the guru becomes a gate. You go through it, but you don't hang onto it. The gate doesn't follow you when you go through it. You don't have to remain dependent on him, even though in the earlier stages you may feel you are becoming dependent. You may think, "What am I going to do if I become so dependent on him?" You forget how dependent you are on money; how dependent you are on power, pleasure, and possessions. You are willing to be dependent on all of those things, yet you don't want to be dependent on a guru who can eventually free you from all dependency. You want to be free. You conveniently forget your other dependencies when it comes to spiritual dependence. Suddenly you want to be independent. But you do not at this stage have the choice of being either dependent or independent; you may only choose what you wish to be dependent upon.

There is a stage where a disciple will be attached to and dependent upon the physical guru. But this attachment, this dependence, is only a stage, only a role to play to go beyond both attachment and dependency. For your growth you eventually learn to attune to the more subtle existence of the guru's energy. You learn to draw directly upon the guru's subtle presence by keeping him in your heart twenty-four hours a day, by thinking of him as the one who inspires you to live a higher life. Then you have grown beyond the bonds of attachment and dependence. You have grown to a level where you can drink the nectar of true spiritual freedom.

**The Need for a Living Master**

You can read as many books as you want, but you will not get true spiritual guidance and inspiration from them. For in-depth realization it is necessary to have a living master. There are more books today than ever before, but there are not proportionally more enlightened people. Books can inspire, but they cannot enlighten. You cannot have a guru who comes to you only through words and writings. Words do not have meaning other than to inspire you. This is the purpose of all writing. Writings cannot show you the truth, they can only direct you. To find truth you must have the direct experience of it. It is the guru's role to give you this experience.

Direction is necessary until you can function with balance and harmony when there is disharmony all around. Until you come to this level, you need the presence of the guru. In the absence of the guru your lower mind will play

66    many tricks to get you off of the higher path. The guru has to constantly guide you through the disappointments and frustrations that often appear on the spiritual path. By ignoring your superficial behavior and seeing your highest potential, the guru turns every situation into a learning experience, a growth experience.

The guru's every action becomes a learning experience for the disciple. As he acts, so he teaches. His manner of sitting, standing, and walking, the way he talks, listens, or keeps silence—each little thing becomes a learning process. Everything is a teaching in the presence of the guru.

When in the presence of the guru, a disciple must be fully conscious, open and aware. At any moment he might receive the spark of enlightenment; he might suddenly understand something he previously heard only with his ears. The disciple must always be on guard for that unexpected moment. Something is done through the guru by his very existence; the disciple need only be ready to receive it. The guru cannot help the disciple who will not accept his help. Those disciples who receive many benefits through a guru are the ones who are open to his teachings. They are ready to receive. The role of a disciple is not only to learn intellectually, but to receive through the heart.

## The Guru-Disciple Relationship

*The guru does not give love. He is love.*

For the disciple to receive from the guru, it is an absolute necessity that love exist between them. You establish a channel of love, a channel of energy, with the guru through your love, dedication, faith, and trust in him. You open yourself to the guru's love. Then you begin to communicate with him regardless of the distance between you. When you love someone, you can communicate without words; but when you hate someone, you can shout and there will be no communication.

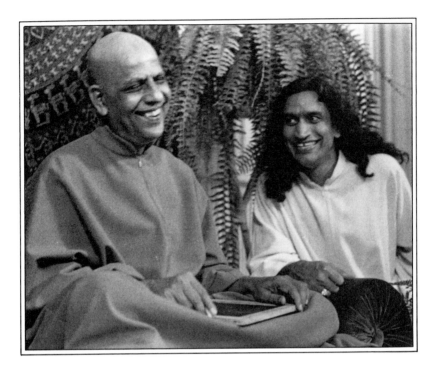

### Trust in the Guru

Trust in the guru is absolutely necessary in order to establish communication. The teachings of the higher path cannot be communicated with words, but only through love and experience. A guru cannot give you a slide show and say, "This is what samadhi is like"; a guru cannot give you a large book and say, "Read this and you will experience samadhi." There is no way a guru can communicate higher experiences with words. These experiences come from beyond the mind, so the mind has no capacity to express them or explain them. Thus it is necessary that communication on the highest level be established. Only love can communicate to the heart without going through the brain. Communication through the brain will inevitably be distorted. Anything you receive through your brain is understood only in terms of the exaggerated needs of the ego. All communication is distorted through the ego's obses-

68    sions and complexes. The ego uses the brain for external communication, while the communication of the heart is inner communication. When you have faith, love, and trust in a guru, you establish an inner energy channel with him. Then his energies automatically begin to flow into you. You will be transformed because your love and respect for the guru allow you to be open to him.

Because the spiritual phenomenon takes place on a subjective level, the guru cannot direct you into it. You can only willingly open yourself to the experience. The objective can be known and learned by words—it can be taught. The subjective can only be communicated when you experience that state of consciousness. You can read all the techniques of swimming and be an expert on swimming theory. That does not insure that you will be able to swim and save your life if you are thrown into a lake. Theory is altogether different from experience. Yoga is not theory; yoga is experience. That is why it is known as the path from the alone to the alone.

Each person experiences something different from their contact with the guru. Each person receives a different energy and experience from the guru, depending on his individual needs. When you begin to love and trust the guru, you establish the energy link of communication so necessary on the spiritual path.

Because all spiritual teachings are experiential, patience, perseverance, and practice are necessary on the part of a disciple. Philosophy can be learned in a short time, but the guru-disciple relationship is one of experience rather than intellectual athletics. Spiritual practices can quickly be explained verbally; no patience or perseverance is required. But to experience spiritual practices, patience and perseverance on the part of the disciple are necessary.

Your ability to receive directly depends on how much faith you have generated in your heart. If a scientist invents something, the entire world can experience it, use it, and receive its benefits. If a yogi reaches the highest, however, he cannot give the benefit of his experience to others unless they are willing to follow with faith, love, and trust. He can not give it, even if he so desires, because spiritual enlightenment is a subjective experience. His willingness to give is not sufficient. Your willingness to receive is equally or more important. If the sun is shining outside but you close all the doors and windows, the sun does not exist for you. You must open the windows and doors to experience the sun's warmth and light.

In order to understand the abstract it is important to have a guru in whom you can place your faith and trust, so he can lead you and guide you. Can you imagine taking a trip in a taxi without knowing if the driver understands where he is going? Or suppose you take a trip to Mt. Everest and you do not know whether you can trust your guide. If you cannot follow him, it is better not to start the journey. But once you have trust in him, you must follow his guidance if you are to benefit from his knowledge.

It is necessary to develop trust and faith in the guru, because your ability to absorb his teachings is dependent on your ability to trust. It is your ability to trust and be open which will allow you to throw away your preconceived ideas, your intellectual doubts and interpretations of experiences. The more trust you have, the more receptive is your heart. This is why the Masters say, "Come to me with an empty cup." Too many thoughts, too many ideas, too many notions, too many insecurities, too many fears keep your cup so full that you cannot receive.

Where does trust begin? Trust begins with experience. A little trust can increase into greater trust by practicing what is given to you. If a doctor gives you medicine and tells you that this is the medicine for your problem, you will have to trust him in order to take it regularly. Then, when the medicine works, you have greater trust in him. But if you didn't trust him in the first place, there would be no place to develop further trust.

A school teacher will draw a line and say, "This is called

70     'one'." If the child says, "No, that is not 'one'," the teaching process is ended. In the beginning the child will have to take it for granted that the teacher is right. In the same way a disciple in his spiritual childhood must follow his guru's teachings.

In every relationship there has to be some trust in the beginning before you establish deeper trust based upon your own experiences. Until you have established your trust based on experience, you will have to trust the external guru. At this stage you cannot command enough inner experience to trust your inner guru. You have to start somewhere, so you start with the external guru. Then when you have direct realizations, your inner guru will be awakened. But your inner guru will not be revealed all at once. You will still have to trust the external guru until you have become fully established in your inner guru.

The relationship between the disciple and the guru is one of intimate trust—trust, open-mindedness, and receptivity. The very nature of the spiritual quest is that of traveling into the unknown. You cannot travel into the unknown unless you have faith and trust in your guide. You will be unable to take even one step forward without faith and trust.

Trust in a guru is trust in yourself. If you trust anybody, you are trusting yourself. It is easier to start with trusting a guru, because he won't confuse or misuse your trust. Trust in a guru is trust in the guru within, trust in your heart. Such trust cannot be taught, it emerges as your need to grow increases. Just as you trust a doctor when you need him, so you will trust a guru when your need to grow is sufficient to command such trust and faith.

On the spiritual path there are many experiences which cannot be used for higher growth unless you have faith and trust in your guru. If you do not have faith and trust, you will run away from these growth experiences. Without trust and faith you cannot grow. You will fall into the same problems over and over again. That is why the basic component of the guru-disciple relationship is trust. People try to interpret spiritual experiences. But these experiences come from another dimension and it is impossible to verbalize them or intellectualize about them. They come from the unknown and can be understood only through experience. That is why faith and trust are necessary. Only trust can allow you to travel fearlessly into the unknown. Whenever you are confronted with the unknown, faith is necessary, trust is necessary.

No matter what you are studying, you have to follow blindly at first. You have to trust your teacher. Trust your guru, follow his guidance thoroughly, and question later. Before you practice there is no room for questioning, because you don't know what to question. Your mind will merely be creating artificial questions with no basis in your experiences. The mind can create questions and the mind can answer questions without making any change in your life. Only after you practice does your question have worth. There can be no opinion without experience. You cannot question what you do not know. Once you have experienced, your questions will be valid. Such questions will help you to grow.

### The Role of Reverence

Reverence is like love with one difference—love is felt for someone on a parallel level, and reverence is felt for one above, one higher. Reverence is love for one who is higher. When there is a loving intimacy towards the higher personality, then there is reverence. This reverence is automatically created around a guru. It is not expected or demanded by the guru, it is a natural outcome of the love and trust of the disciple.

Such reverence is necessary for you to receive from a spiritual teacher. A teacher cannot teach if the students are sitting up higher than the teacher. The energy exchange does not facilitate spiritual teaching. The spiritual teacher

72 has to sit on a higher level, because energy flows from the higher to the lower. If you try to stay at a higher level, you will remain as dry as the mountains, while the valleys are green and filled with lakes. This is because valleys receive water from the mountains. In the same way the disciple receives from the guru by dropping his ego and being humble, open, and receptive to what the guru has to give. That is why bowing is necessary—necessary for the disciple, not for the guru. The disciple must understand what it means to sit at a lower level and be totally receptive to the guru. If you want to become a mountain, you must start out as a valley, you must accept that you are a valley. But when there is a true relationship of giving and receiving, there comes a time when you are beyond both the mountains and the valleys.

### The Disciple's Love

A guru is not his physical form. You may start by loving his physical form, but that is not where your love will end. There comes a time when you transcend the physical form of the guru. There comes a time when his physical form dissolves as you truly experience the depth and beauty of inner love. It is not the love for the guru that is most significant. Your heart is opening through love for him—that is the significant phenomenon. When your heart opens, it excludes none. It can encompass all.

The love for a guru begins with his physical form because you are used to acknowledging love through the physical form. That's the way it begins, but that is not the way it ends.

A guru will accept your love even if you love his physical form. That is a beginning. From there he can transform your love into a higher love. If your love starts that way it is fine, as long as you love him. Let your love be so exclusive that nothing remains in your mind but love. Then the transformation will take place. The whole secret of growing on the spiritual path is this: love transforms. When love becomes so loud and clear that everything subsides under it, you have progressed tremendously. Physical love has no outlet with a guru. You will be forced to transform it into a more refined, spiritual love. Then, even if you leave him physically, you will never leave his love. His love will continue to work through you and permeate your entire being. In the initial stages, love him in any way you want, but always remain aware.

All the guru wants is your spiritual growth. He sees this as the real application of love. All he wants is for you to throw away your weaknesses and burn them in his love. The stronger the fire of your love, the stronger will be your capacity to burn all personal desires and selfishness and be purified in that fire of love.

This love relationship is unlike any other relationship you have ever seen or experienced. You cannot compare it to any relationship you have had before. Ordinarily love between two people is conditional love. But the love of a guru is unconditional. The guru wants you to love him so you can love yourself, so you can awaken the divine within you.

If you love a guru, you love yourself. You have seen something worthwhile within yourself and you are using the guru as a reflector. That is all the guru wants to be—a reflector, a mirror of your love. You cannot love yourself directly because you are so close to yourself that you cannot see yourself. But you can love yourself through the guru.

The guru takes you away from yourself so you can see yourself. He does this by taking the accent off of you and putting it on him. By loving the guru you are indirectly serving yourself. So love for a guru allows you to be objective toward yourself. If you cannot be objective, you cannot love.

You love the external guru exclusively to establish contact with him. Then you begin to receive what he has to offer. But for you to receive you must give your heart wholly to him. As you grow in your love for the guru, your

74    energy will be transformed into his. Those who love a guru are automatically connected to his flow of energy. Then many problems are washed away.

This love is an exchange of energy. No matter who you love, the qualities of that loved one will begin to flow into you unconsciously and instantly, depending on how much you love that person. This is why it is very important to be discriminating where you place your love.

If you do not have a love relationship with your guru, it will be very difficult for you to learn from him. But once you love him he doesn't have to teach you verbally. You at once adopt his methods of talking, thinking, and living. If you do not love him, there is no basis on which to establish the energy contact. The close contact of love plays an important role in the communication of the higher and more subtle levels of love. Love cannot be communicated verbally, it must be experienced.

You must do everything on your part to intensify your love and trust for the guru by removing yourself from any distractions of company or books which create doubt within your mind. Remove all thoughts that create distrust and doubt. There is no situation or person on earth whom you cannot doubt for some reason if you so desire. Even Christ was doubted. The guru can answer your questions, but he can never answer your doubt. A question can be answered, but a doubt can only be dropped.

Your love for the guru not only helps you, it also helps the guru to help you. It helps the love of the guru grow stronger so he can love you. Trust in a guru gives him greater strength to trust. Then he redistributes this love and trust to others. Love is like the fragrance of a flower. How can the flower keep its fragrance? It is impossible. It is the flower's very nature to release its fragrance into the air and please many noses. By loving a guru you begin to love all, but your love must begin with one person before it can go out to many.

## Qualities of a Disciple

It is not merely the guru who is playing the important role, but also the disciple. It is said, "When the disciple is ready, the guru will appear." But if the disciple is not ready and the guru appears physically, it doesn't mean the guru has appeared. The guru will appear only to that person who has established a contact of love energy with the guru. Only then will the energy begin to flow. So the guru never inflicts his energy without the other person's cooperation. Even God does not take that privilege. God helps only those who help themselves. It begins with you. You will have to be open and receptive in order to receive the guru. The disciple must be ready, he must be open, and he must be wholehearted in his desire for growth.

To be generated, energy must have positive and negative poles. This is what happens between a guru and a disciple. They create opposite poles—the disciples demand and the guru becomes alert. Like two wings of a bird, the guru and disciple enhance each other. the guru receives energy as he gives energy to you. The more energy you give him, the more he will have to give to others in need and the more he will have to give to you when you are in need.

### The Role of the Guru in Shaktipat Kundalini Yoga

On coming into the presence of a true guru, the person who is ready and open begins to feel waves of bliss. He experiences something new, something unusual that he doesn't understand. He feels very different. Involuntary motions begin to occur. He may feel heat or cold, or sometimes he will experience crying, laughing, or shaking for no apparent reason. All the while he feels ecstatic. These experiences are the result of the transference of psychic energy, known as Shakti, from the guru to the disciple.

After this transference, the disciple suddenly experiences many changes in his life. These changes occur as the guru's energy, active within the disciple, begins an auto-

76  matic process of purification on all levels—physical, mental, emotional, and spiritual.

### Effects of Shaktipat

After Shaktipat the guru's energy enters the disciple and accomplishes changes within the disciple in minutes that otherwise would have taken many years to accomplish. The flow of energy within the disciple is reversed. It is no longer externalized, but becomes focused within at higher levels of consciousness. The disciple is quickly transformed.

The spontaneous merging of energies that occurs during Shaktipat at once begins to promote a great magnetic attraction in the disciple for the guru. Psychic communication is established and the disciple gradually begins to merge and vibrate with the guru's energy, thus establishing a mystical tie that provides constant guidance and protection on the higher path. As the energy of the guru actually enters the disciple an attitude of love spontaneously arises in the disciple for the guru. The tie of direct, inner communication is established. Only love can convey what the tongue cannot carry, what language cannot express. This love is a spontaneous occurrence on the path of Shaktipat Kundalini Yoga.

When this energy is awakened, you may go through difficulties or frustrations of varying degrees as the energy accomplishes its task of purification. This purification process is different for each individual, because no two individuals are alike in their bodies, minds, emotions, and past or future hopes. You may go through emotional purification which may cause disappointments and temporary depressions. This happens because deep-seated blocks are being released. As these blocks go out they throw their aroma around you, just as a garbage can smells bad when you clean it. It has to smell bad if you are to get rid of the garbage, but that doesn't mean there is anything wrong. You are merely emptying the garbage. You are stripping

yourself of many difficulties of your past—physical, emotional, and psychological—which have become an integral
part of your personality. This can be a painful process, but
by the grace of the guru and through your trust in his
guidance, you realize this is just a cleansing phenomenon.
Then you quickly pass through it.

At such times of cleansing and purification the need
for a guru is more necessary than at any other time because
of the nature and speed of the purification process. It is at
these times that a disciple must have complete dedication,
love, and trust. The ability of the guru to help is important,
but the openness of the disciple to receive that help is
equally as important. On the path of Shaktipat Kundalini
Yoga the progress of a disciple is quick only if the disciple
has trust and faith in the guru. Because the purification
process progresses so quickly, many physical, emotional,
and mental upheavels may be brought about. At such times
the more faith, trust, and surrender a disciple has, the
more quickly he passes through these temporary difficulties
and the faster is his progress on the spiritual path.

To have a Shakti experience is not in itself enough to
make you grow. You may receive strong energy and have
experiences similar to Shakti in the presence of well-known
personalities, spiritual teachers, or in the Pentecostal
Church. These experiences are spiritual in nature, but they
must be understood further through the guidance of a
guru. Just as electricity is useless and often destructive
when unchanneled in the form of lightening, Shakti, when
it is not channeled through the pure medium of a guru, is of
little value for spiritual growth. When harnessed and har-
monized through a medium, electricity provides us with
light. In the same way the guru is the medium through
which the disciple learns how to channel Shakti so it may
bring inner bliss and peace.

When you receive Shakti from a guru, he facilitates
your growth very quickly by providing you with a situation
in which your love and trust can grow. But you must re-

78    main open. The seed is no more potent than the ground on which it falls. The ground must be fertile if the seed is to grow. A disciple must be spiritually fertile to insure the growth of the seeds of knowledge and wisdom sown by the guru.

## The Ashram: Home of the Guru

The ashram is a specially designed spiritual home which provides growth for the disciple at each stage of his development. It is an expression of the guru's energy which snowballs and grows larger and stronger as it circulates among the resident disciples. In this way the ashram provides a means for spreading the guru's energy of love.

The ashram is the home of your spiritual family. It provides a surrounding where you are loved by the guru and his disciples, in which you are accepted unconditionally. The love of the guru and his disciples is given freely to all. The love-filled atmosphere of the ashram opens the heart of the spiritual seeker who then becomes a receptacle of love.

The home of the guru, the ashram, is also a home for spiritual seekers who wish to grow through serving the guru and practicing his teaching on an everyday basis. For one who wishes to grow spiritually the proper surrounding and the proper external guidance are absolute necessities. By providing both, the ashram creates a situation in which inner as well as external harmony may be achieved. The ashram is a situation in which the teachings of the guru can immediately be experienced. It is through this experience that rapid growth and deep inner changes are achieved.

The ashram is a reflection, a mirror image of the guru. It is through the ashram that his teachings are most deeply communicated. By actually experiencing what cannot be communicated verbally, the disciple can fully understand the guru's wisdom and love. Truth can be discovered only through experience.

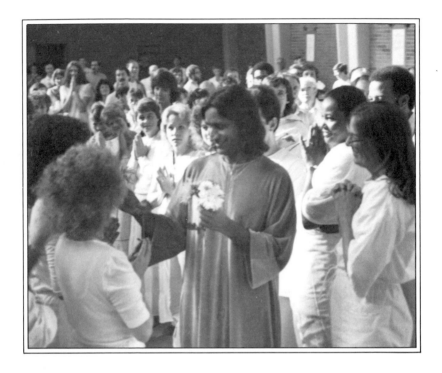

## Surrender and Discipline

*Surrender can only be called surrender if it leads you back to the source.*

There are barriers which keep the energy from flowing smoothly between the inner and external guru. As soon as you surrender, however, your inner and external guru will merge. You will no longer have tension, worry, fear, or emotional problems. But you must surrender. Surrendering means living in the present. You cannot stop worrying if you live in the future. The future happens only with insecurity; the future is always unknown. You can only dream about tomorrow. When you project that tomorrow will be better, you are not facing the present. You are holding onto your dreams and ignoring what is happening now. As long as you live in the hope of the future, you cannot surrender. Surrender shatters your dreams of the future

80 and brings you into the present, enabling you to be happy. Happiness does not exist in the future; happiness exists only in the present. By surrendering you destroy the root of all sickness and problems, psychological, emotional, and physiological. You give up your fears. You give up your worries.

Surrender means total trust and acceptance of the present. This acceptance of the present is trust in the guru, trust in his guidance. But unless you trust yourself first, you cannot trust the guru. Paradoxically, it is the guru who helps you trust and accept yourself, thereby helping you to trust the guru more completely.

The guru takes you step by step, not asking you to believe everything in the beginning. If you stay with him, however, your trust and faith in him will develop spontaneously. The guru does not ask you to trust for himself, but so he can help you give everything to God; so he can help you drop all of your attachments—your false identity and fears, your mental struggling and your changing emotions. All the guru will ask of you is that you give him your problems. That's all he wants.

People fear that a guru will take everything away from them. Yet they don't define clearly what they have to offer. What do you have to offer, other than your problems? As Bapuji says, in his bhajan (devotional song) addressed to the Lord, "What can I offer you that is not already yours? All that I can offer are my problems, that is all I have created. What else can I offer? When I look around I see all creation is yours. All that I have created is my problems." Your problems are the best gift you can give your guru. He wants nothing else but that you surrender all of your ego. As you surrender your weaknesses a new dawn, a new light will suddenly come into your life. Surrender is the path of forgetting—forgetting your problems. You hand them to the guru and you forget them. They are now his responsibility. The disciple, who is asleep, surrenders, and the guru, who is awake, takes the responsibility.

Surrender means surrendering the results of your actions. Neither success nor failure concern you. You do not become careless, but you do become worryless. This is the true meaning of surrender. Total surrender is necessary so your mind may be totally free from all tensions, fears, and frustrations of ego.

Listen with your heart; listen with your past experiences. Trust what your experience says by truly understanding what life has given you in the way you have lived. Sincerely ask if that is what you want from life. If the answer is no, if you haven't received what you want, what you are really looking for, then the guru is there. He can guide you, he can lead you, he can help you, he can protect you, he can do everything for you if you surrender. But it is necessary to give up all desires, preconceived ideas, and the competitive spirit you once had. Those things don't work on the spiritual path. In the outer world you have to fight to receive what you want. In the spiritual world you have to surrender. These worlds work by two different standards.

To surrender you must keep your energy high. Only then can you give up ego. This is the secret. You have to have a lot of energy, a lot of strength, a lot of peace to give up ego. In order to give up ego, in order to surrender, you have to function at peak performance in everything you do. When you do everything well, a very high energy is released from within. When that energy is released, you suddenly trust everybody because you trust yourself. As soon as you begin to trust yourself, the guru within gives more trust to the external guru, thereby establishing the contact of energy between your inner and outer guru. As the energy circulates between you and your external guru, you begin to feel much love for him.

Your true love for your guru is true surrender. Don't expect anything. Just surrender to whatever happens. Practical surrender to a guru will produce real surrender. You practice what the guru says and as a result you naturally have greater and greater surrender. Your mind will no longer fluctuate. You will be in balance.

With the death of the wavering mind you go into a transcendental state. But to do this you must remain centered. Being centered means not identifying with your whims, your changing desires, expectations, hopes, and dreams. This process of centering is called surrender.

## Freedom and Discipline

Surrender is possible only after you establish a certain form of discipline. This discipline will eventually take you beyond discipline, because discipline results in surrender. In surrender there is a stage of discipline before real surrender comes. With surrender comes freedom. Freedom means discipline. The result of discipline is freedom. But first you must work on discipline. Don't worry about surrender in the beginning. Put all of your energy into discipline and then surrender will come naturally.

If discipline is ignored in the beginning, the false concept of liberty, of freedom, will become a license for wrong habits. Such freedom brings self-destruction, self-deception, and greater bondage. It is like the river that merges with the ocean and then tells the other rivers that their banks are shackles, self-imposed and unnecessary. Such a sermon is a fallacy for the rivers who have not yet met their father, the ocean. If the rivers give up their banks of discipline prematurely, before meeting the ocean, they will spread and destroy fields and towns. Then they will dry up and disappear in utter self-destruction before reaching their goal.

Freedom in the hands of a fool can be fatal. In the earlier stages of spiritual practices the spiritual child needs loving guidance, loving care and surroundings, and loving discipline. The crib for a child is a discipline. Such confinement is needed to protect the child physically as he has not yet developed sufficient discrimination to protect himself. As soon as he develops discrimination he will be ready to handle physical freedom. But then he will need to be disciplined on other levels where he has not yet developed discrimination. In the same way the guru disciplines the disciple only to bring him to the state of surrender. Surrender means practicing the disciplines given by the guru. Discipline leads to surrender. Surrender leads to eventual freedom. Discipline is the key to freedom.

True love for your guru is not saying, "I love you, I love you." The real way to love your guru is to practice what he teaches, because a true guru is his teachings. Be very firm in the disciplines given by the guru. Then you will have faith, trust, and experience which are beyond the verbal level. A guru is not independent of his teachings. You can invite his presence only by practicing his teachings. The guru and his teachings are one. If you ignore the teachings, you are ignoring the guru.

## Growing into Surrender

This state of surrender comes as the result of non-attachment, selflessness, and total dedication to a higher purpose. When you put all these ingredients together, they automatically create surrender. The moment you surrender you will begin to change in a profound manner. Your heart will experience rest and peace. But you must totally let go and have no personal desires, no selfish motives. With this surrender you become a part of the psychic root system of the guru. You accept him and you accept the growth you want through him. In this state of surrender the disciple is linked to the direct source of the guru's deeper knowledge. Growth takes place in a higher, psychic dimension.

If you don't have surrender, you can develop it gradually by practicing willful disciplines. Different individuals have different amounts of surrender and will. It is good to work with both surrender and will, because we all are a mixture of the two. There are a few stages that work with will before you come to the stage of surrender. Both quali-

84      ties, will and surrender, are necessary.

But you can surrender only when you do everything in the best possible way. In order to surrender, your heart must be clear. In your heart you must be absolutely clean. You must be doing everything in the right way, working hard, working lovingly, without guilt. Guilt paves the way for anger, hatred, jealousy and fear. These are the blocks to surrender.

As you surrender you begin to taste the real fruit of surrender, which is responsibility. Responsibility means you have the ability to respond to any given situation in the best possible way. Only when you live in the present can you do this. When you live in the future, there is fear and your ability to respond deteriorates. To respond properly you cannot live in the future, you cannot be attached to results which lie in the future. Attachment to results brings fear and worry. Where there is fear, there is no love; where there is no love, there is no compassion. Compassion exists in non-attachment. The more non-attached you become, the more universal you become; the more attached, the more limited you become. As soon as you become attached, your ability to respond is lowered. Only in non-attachment is there true love. Then devotion assumes a depth that allows no space for fear. That is why there is so much emphasis on devotion, dedication, and surrender. If you have surrender, then the guru can work for you. God can work for you. Then there is nothing you cannot do. Nothing can overpower you. You are always protected. But your protection is directly proportional to your surrender, your dedication.

If you depend on your selfish ego, you are responsible for your actions. You must answer for them. But when you surrender to God and guru, they are obliged to take care of you and they do so. Then God and guru become your protectors and your guides.

When you surrender, you want nothing. All is given to the guru, all is dedicated to the guru. Then you become fearless. Surrender at once provides you with fearlessness, because you want nothing. You know that the guru is taking care of you. There is nothing in life you cannot face. No obstacle or challenge can keep you from inner peace, because you are no longer responsible. It is done for you by the guru.

## The Stages of the Guru's Discipline

Eventually the guru and the disciple become one. They merge into the ocean of no discipline. Time passes, and the discipline grows milder and milder as the disciple's ability to respond in a spontaneously surrendered manner increases. As this ability increases, there is no longer the need for discipline.

As the disciple passes through various stages of growth on the spiritual path, he requires specific disciplines given by the guru and gradually becomes more capable of handling freedom and responsibility.

In the earliest stage of growth the guru has to take loving care of the disciple to protect him against many hazards, as the disciple has not yet developed discrimination. In the earliest stage the guru is a mother to the disciple. When the child throws tantrums, does not know how to eat, how to use the bathroom, or how to clean himself, the mother considers it a special privilege and a great joy to take care of the child in every respect. The mother gladly shares her own body, her own life with the newly conceived child in her womb. She looks forward to the birth of the new baby in spite of the inexpressible pain she will have to go through at the time of birth. The ecstasy of having her own energies molded into a new life gives her the strength, power, and faith to face any fear and pain. In the same way the guru is also always glad to go through the pain and problems of giving spiritual birth to a disciple.

Such a spiritual child needs the protection and motherly love of the guru. As he grows, however, he soon needs

86 firm guidance and discipline. At this stage the guru teaches the disciple by assuming the role of a father, a disciplinarian. When the disciple grows through that stage, he becomes mature enough to have brotherly discipline and then he graduates into friendly discipline. Finally the guru and disciple merge into oneness—as the river merges into the ocean of no discipline, existence beyond bonds, infinite oneness, and ecstasy of union.

The guru is all, mother, father, brother, friend. He takes you through every stage on the path. He takes you all the way to God, beginning from the motherly care he gives to generate your spiritual birth, through all the stages of growth and hazards, problems, and difficulties. It is a tough journey, but the guru gladly takes that responsibility. He becomes the vehicle through which you can be purified.

The oldest prayer to the guru says:

*Thou art my mother, my father thou art,*
*Thou art my brother, my friend thou art,*
*Thou art my knowledge, my wealth thou art,*
*Thou art my all, my God of Gods thou art.*

## Attuning to the Guru Throughout the Day

*True love for the guru is practice of his teachings.*

### Guru Seva: Selfless Service

Kundalini meditation is the process of emptying the cup of ego, selfish desires, and self-destructive habit patterns. For this catharsis of karma (the accumulated result of past thoughts, emotions, and actions which influences our thoughts, emotions, and actions in the present) to take place most effectively and efficiently, the disciple must surrender to the guru. This surrender gradually develops within the disciple as he gives of himself—his time, his talents, his energies, his ego, his desires—both externally and internally, in the process known as guru seva. Guru seva is work performed as selfless service to the guru, in the spirit of Karma Yoga (the yoga of non-attached action). Actions performed as guru seva become an expression of love rather than ego. Receiving the disciple's services is not the need of the guru. Giving service, however, is the need of the disciple. By giving the guru a gift the disciple can, with a free conscience, be open to receive the guru's teachings. In this way guru seva psychologically opens the disciple to receive the grace of the guru and makes possible further and deeper commitment and faith. Thus service leads to surrender, and, as surrender deepens, love grows. Without surrender, love is not possible.

When a new disciple first comes to a guru, he is established in discipleship by a special ceremony called Mantra Initiation, or by Shaktipat Initiation. As he begins to follow the disciplines given by the guru, he executes all of his worldly duties as an offering of worship and service to the guru. All actions being offered to the guru, the disciple performs them in the most efficient and creative manner possible, using all the imagination and energy available to him at any given time. He discharges all duties and responsibilities, whether at work, at home, or at the ashram, with love. He performs every action as if he were in the presence of his guru, as if he were doing it just for his guru. He renounces all attachments to his work along with all results arising from his work. By remaining attuned to his guru's love and energy, he begins to purify his ego and lower desires.

It is highly recommended that a disciple serve his guru with all his possessions, power, and energy, so that the energy which is trapped and consumed by his attachments to power and possessions can be released and made available for his spiritual growth in love, for love, and through love. This love begins as service to the external guru, but it grows to become service and love for the guru within, eventually extending to service and love for all humanity.

## 88 The Guru's Service

The guru accepts the disciple's service without attachment or expectation, as an act of true love and service to all seekers who approach him for guidance. In the earlier stages of the disciple's growth he willingly allows the disciple to believe that he needs the disciple's help, knowing very well that the disciple must first give of himself before he is truly open to receive the guru's wisdom. At this stage the guru does not discourage the disciple from giving, even if the disciple gives with egotistical motivation. The disciple's service to the guru, even if it is done with ego in the beginning, is necessary to help the disciple establish an energy contact with the guru. Once the disciple has given of himself, he automatically begins to be transformed in an effortless, invisible, and very subtle manner. The disciple's store of karma is exhausted and he is gradually emptied of ego and selfish desires through service and surrender with love. Knowing this, the guru may allow the disciple to think that it is the need of the guru to receive the services of the disciple. Sometimes, if it is necessary, the guru even helps fatten the disciple's ego, well aware at each stage that he is going to butcher it mercilessly one day.

Just as children, up to a certain age, need to grow in ego, so must the disciple if he is to eventually discover the consequences of ego. He will then know that his ego is the source of his suffering and realize the need to drop it. Being aware of this fact, the guru first focuses his attention on loving the disciple, regardless of how he acts. In order to serve the disciple, the guru gladly lowers his own consciousness and vibrates at the disciple's energy level in order to communicate with him. Hence the guru seems to be catering to the disciple's ego, but there is no other way to help him. If the fork lift wants to lift the load off the ground, the fork will have to lower itself to the bottom level of the load to lift. So also the guru brings himself to mundane, worldly details and dealings, in a totally detached manner, in order to lift the disciple above his destructive, egotistical habits. Through every action the guru is teaching the disciple. Through every action the guru is a guide, an instrument for the growth of the disciple.

## Attuning to the Guru's Presence

Once you surrender to the guru, you are no longer the victim of self-destructive habits and desires. Regardless of what happens to you—success or failure, happiness or unhappiness, joy or sorrow—you surrender to the guru and remain established in guru seva. Through service and surrender with love, you strengthen your attunement to the guru's energy. As you dwell upon the guru in each daily activity, your life is transformed into one of continuous meditation. As you constantly draw upon the guru's love and energy, the guru begins to work within you, washing away all of your impurities and transforming you on all levels of being.

When you love someone, you can be transformed into him. If you attune your energies to that person, you are establishing a subtle channel so you may draw energy from him. When you love your guru, you love his teachings. You practice them almost effortlessly. Then your guru begins to work through you. He is with you, not in his body, but in the essence of his teachings.

How can you remain attuned to your guru's energy and teachings? You remain attuned by remaining relaxed. Throughout the day, remain physically calm, mentally calm. Remove all desires, comparisons, mental cravings. Whenever you think of your guru, instantly become relaxed. Be totally open, wanting nothing, expecting nothing. As soon as stillness pervades, you will know that there is God within you and you will feel the presence of the guru. Then continue with whatever work you were doing.

Once you learn to remain established in the guru you

90     can accomplish any amount of work at peak performance and still be relaxed. All problems, all difficulties which you habitually face—the depression, fear, tension, tiredness, feelings of inadequacy—all will gradually be resolved because now the guru's energy is inside you and working through you. But there is a requirement—that you remain calm, remain relaxed, remain attuned and in harmony with the guru. As often as possible tell yourself, "I want nothing. I want to be nothing. I brought nothing with me, nor will I take anything when I go. I want to accomplish nothing for myself. I give my life to God and my guru."

In those moments of wanting nothing, the real things in life happen. For when you truly expect nothing, you will be transformed. It can happen in an instant. So remain calm, remain attuned, and know that you are protected. That means trusting the guru, that means attunement to the guru. The real attunement to the guru is this: remaining centered and at peace. That is the greatest service, the greatest love you can give. Because all the guru wants is your happiness and growth.

### Receiving the Guru's Guidance

Continuous inner contact constructs a channel between the master and the disciple. The more the inner contact, the stronger is this channel of energy transference. Then you can desire guidance and you will receive it instantly, effortlessly. All you have to do is think of your guru and he will be there to guide you and protect you.

Visualize yourself sitting in front of your guru. Invite him into your heart. Ask for his guidance. Ask, "What would you do in this situation?" As you ask, your inner guru will begin to merge into your external guru. Then a unique phenomenon will take place. The guidance will flow naturally through you. You will begin to experience the guru's love and energy with such a deep sensitivity that a new awareness will begin to dawn spontaneously within you. You will no longer have to ask for direction. You will be subtly guided all the time.

But you must become a pure channel so the energy is not filtered through the impurities of ego and selfish desires. Establish the channel, but purify it at the same time. Until you become pure, test your inner guidance by logic, experience, and common sense. If you are following the true guidance of a guru, you will never be in a situation that will make you tense, fearful or restless.

There is no limit to the energy you can receive by attuning to the guru. You will never feel tired, you will never feel confused or afraid, as long as you draw on his presence. You will become a fountain of energy as the energy of the guru flows through you. This is how you transform your energy of love into higher growth.

Establish firm contact with your inner guru by attuning to your external guru. As you follow the inner guidance, you will be transformed. This is not worship in the conventional sense, it is practical worship, designed to lead you to the highest consciousness.

The guru begins to construct your channel of energy with him by giving you a mantra. A mantra is a sound or rhythmic sequence of sounds which, when correctly intoned, releases potent energies within the person chanting. Perceived by yogis in the state of Samadhi or Universal Consciousness, mantras are used to go beyond the realm of words, to destroy the veil of separation and allow you to be reunited with your true blissful self. When you chant the mantra given by your guru, you draw upon the accumulated strength of all masters who have attained enlightenment by using that particular mantra.

Chanting guru mantra is a most effective way to contact the guru's energy. As you continually chant guru mantra, you will constantly collect the guru's energy. As you continue to chant guru mantra and build up a reservoir of energy, all problems, big and small, can be dissolved. Repeat the mantra constantly. By chanting the mantra when you

92 are not in difficulty, you will build its power within you so it can more potently help you in difficult situations. As you continuously accumulate the guru's energy, through the repetition of guru mantra, you will be able to call upon it whenever you are in difficulty. Then the guru will truly be with you, not just in times of difficulty, but also in times of joy. He will truly reside in your heart as you reside in his.

## The Guru: A Postscript

Through love the guru transforms and awakens the dormant energies within the disciple. Through love the disciple realizes his full potential; he awakens to his full beauty; he perceives his unity with the Father. The guru provides the link between God, the Father, and the disciple, His child. Our attachments bind us to the darkness of the earth. The guru allows us to see the divine light of God and opens us to receive it.

The heart of spiritual growth is the guru. He constantly guides and inspires the disciple to attain a higher level of consciousness. He teaches, not only with words, but by his every action. His life becomes a teaching for the dedicated disciple.

He fulfills all roles and relationships for the disciple. Gently he guides the novice seeker. When firm discipline or tender love is needed, he is ready to provide it. Whatever the disciple needs, the guru is ready to give. He gives of his love and his life selflessly, asking nothing in return. The guru's total non-attachment allows the disciple to follow the guru's guidance and uncover his true identity.

To be a disciple is to experience love in its purest form—with non-attachment, with total compassion. To be a guru is to give love unconditionally with non-expectation. The guru-disciple relationship is one of the lover and the beloved.

# God Is Energy

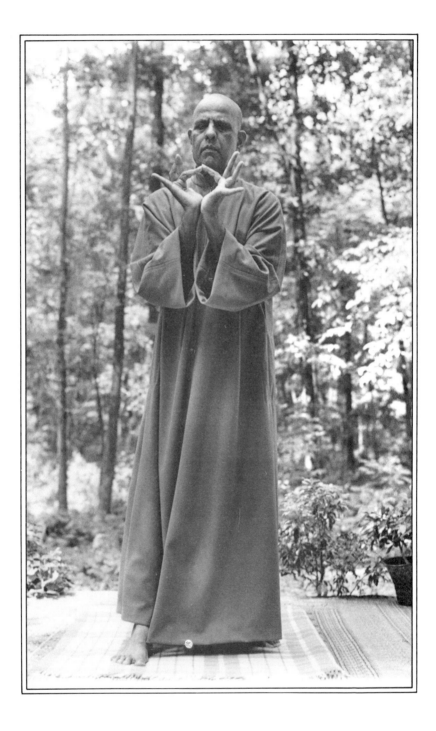

## Paths to the Divine

There are two types of religion: one in which God is believed to be outside man and another in which God is believed to be within man. On the first religious path, God is described as an entity descending from above, from heaven. Heaven is up in the sky, beyond man's reach and remote from his existence. The main method of communication with God on this path is prayer.

The person who follows this path believes that God's grace will save him, remove his pain and suffering and restore him to a distant and future heaven. He believes himself to be totally dependent on God and relies completely on the compassion and mercy of God. "Thy will be done, O Lord, and not mine," is his prayer. This person's journey begins with surrender. His path is the path of prayer and surrender—the path of Bhakti Yoga. Christianity and Islam are clear examples of religions which fall into this category.

The second type of path teaches that God exists within man. He is not remote from man's existence nor far from his reach. He is as close as man's very breath. The purpose of following such a path is to uncover the God who already exists within, while the purpose of following the path of prayer is to gain the favor of a God who exists outside. The path that believes God to be outside solicits His grace through prayer; the path that believes God to be within strives to uncover Him through meditation. Prayer speaks to God without; meditation listens to God within. The man of prayer says, "My Lord, come to me. Do this for me." The man of meditation, on the other hand, says "Aham Brahmasmi" (I am the Brahman—I am God) and "Tat Twam Asi" (Thou art That).

When the actual presence of God is believed to reside within the body of man, the body is considered to be the temple of God. As such, care of the body is stressed to a greater degree than it is on religious paths which believe

96    God to be an entity separate from man. Yoga has designed
an elaborate system which considers care of the body to be
an integral part of spiritual growth. In most religions, spiritual growth has nothing to do with the body. The body is
ignored and, in some cases, even shunned. This is not the
case in yoga. Spiritual practices on the yogic path concern
themselves initially with the tangible body, the body which
man experiences and feels. They gradually lead man to
understand the more subtle levels of his being. The physical practices are designed to affect the glands, muscles,
nerves, tissues, cells and organs of the body as well as the
body's major systems.

The body, which is seen as the temple of God, is also
recognized as the instrument through which oneness with
God is achieved. It is like a bowl which is full of milk. The
bowl is useful to contain the milk which is not yet drunk.
When the milk is gone, however, the bowl has served its
purpose and is no longer useful. In like manner, the body is
useful to contain the energy of God within man. When man
has fully realized God, the body is no longer useful. It is a
tool and not an end in itself—it is the temple of God, but it is
not God Himself.

Kundalini Yoga is based upon this approach. Thus the
yogi on the Kundalini path begins with the body and gradually progresses to the deeper spiritual practices of meditation. He applies his will as well as his reason and logic to his
search for God. In contrast with the practitioner on the
path of prayer, who begins with surrender, the yogi's journey begins largely through the path of will. The beauty of
the path of will is that the journey starts where the majority of aspirants are—it starts with what they can readily
understand, communicate, experience and accept. It begins
with the known, the external, the tangible and the concrete. The practitioner can be sure of what is happening
when he deals with the body. He can feel and see the results
of his practices. Thus the path of will is well-suited to the
Western mind, which responds best to what is external,

tangible and concrete.

The practitioner on the path of will, however, eventually comes to a stage in which he must let go of his will and allow the inner workings of the God within him to direct his progress. This letting go is called surrender. In eight-limbed Ashtanga Yoga, the first six steps, that of Yama (abstention from wrong-doing), Niyama (moral observances), Asana (posture), Pranayama (control of breath), Pratyahara (withdrawal of the mind from sense objects), and Dharana (concentration) belong to the path of will. The last two, Dhyana (meditation) and Samadhi (merger into the center of the Self) belong to the path of surrender. When the disciple arrives at the stage of surrender, he can no longer progress by using his will. His will, in fact, becomes a hindrance to him. At this stage, faith, trust and surrender are necessary to make continued growth possible. The faith and trust needed by the disciple, however, are now available to him as a result of his prior, willful practices.

The Kundalini path progresses from the known to the unknown. When your journey begins with a God of whom you know nothing, it starts with the abstract, with what you are not. Such a search is a journey from the unknown to the unknown. To make such a journey is difficult for the man of logic, the man of reason and will. If you have the faith to surrender to the unknown, to jump into the unknown, then the path of surrender is valid at the very beginning of the search. If you do not have a sufficient amount of faith, however, you will find it difficult to use this approach. Such is the predicament of the average Western practitioner of traditional, faith-oriented religion.

The devotee, the follower of the path of prayer and faith, folds his hands and prays to the Father for His grace—and waits. The yogi, who believes the dormant aspect of God to be within himself, goes through various disciplines to awaken the energy of God, known as Shakti, within him. He acts. He begins with willful, conscious practices. This difference in approach does not mean that

98    prayer can be used only by those who believe God to be outside themselves. It also plays a useful role on the path of will, for prayer, in some form, can be and is used by all paths and in every religion. Prayer without attention to and care of the body, however, is an abstract prayer—a useless prayer.

If the person who prays to God lacks total faith and abiding trust, he will become vague in his belief of God. If he further ignores his body and condemns it, he will fail to see the power of God functioning through his body. He will tend to reject and separate the apparently lower forces of the body from the higher forces of God. As a result, it will become psychologically difficult for him to believe that the kingdom of heaven is within, that God can express Himself through man.

People of this belief unconsciously treat the body and its forces as devilish. They see that the sensual pleasures of lust and passion are so powerful that they distract the aspirant from the higher path. The saying "the Spirit is willing, but the flesh is weak" is correct. The body can indeed be an obstacle, but, when ignored, it becomes a greater obstacle. Only through understanding, study and proper care can man permanently transcend any obstacle, including the body.

When man accepts the presence of Divine energy in each center of his body, even in the traditionally condemned sex center, he truly realizes that God is everywhere. Thus he begins to see God's presence manifesting through every aspect of his being. He realizes that God is energy, that God is neutral in nature like electricity, which can be used to help man or to hurt him. It is man's choice to use this energy of God within him for higher growth or to misuse it for his own selfish gain and sensual pleasure. Yogis realize this fact and, through Hatha and Kundalini Yoga techniques, they purify the body and mind, thereby internalizing their so-called sensual energy for use as a vehicle to achieve expanded states of consciousness. Thus the very sensual energy which is regarded as man's greatest obstacle on the path of prayer becomes the means for higher growth when God is accepted as existing within man through the understanding available in Kundalini Yoga.

When man sees God within himself, he easily recognizes His presence within everyone and everything that surrounds him. He finds it easy to be at one with God. When man sees God as outside and above himself, he experiences a separation, a psychological dichotomy of good and bad, high and low, a dichotomy between heaven and the hell of the flesh, between all earthly beings and their remote Creator. He fails to understand the implications of his belief that God is omnipotent, omniscient and omnipresent. If God is everywhere, He is also in the body.

Because he believes God to be other than himself, man unconsciously condemns himself and the world in order to love a God who is other than himself and the world. He feels he is nobody, that he is weak because of his human flesh. Because he has separated himself from God by separating his body from God, he suffers a tremendous amount of guilt and shame. He feels only God's grace can save him, and God's grace can save him—but if man does not have total faith and trust, he will not be able to receive this grace. At the same time he will fail to do anything on his own, with his own will, to transform himself. If such a man does not receive God's grace or establish some sort of communication with the Divine, he has nothing. He has neither a way to contact grace nor the concrete methods of working through the body.

The path of prayer is difficult for the average person to follow because it is based on faith. Man lives in an age of reason, an age of scientific explanation. The average person who wants logic and experiential proof of the truth of teachings finds it hard to accept a religion through faith alone. For this reason, the path of prayer and faith is difficult for modern man to accept. Yoga, on the other hand, is easily followed and well-accepted because it uses logic and reasoning as tools to acquire faith. It provides unique ben-

100 efits to many people because it does not require either faith or will alone, but provides approaches which are suited to people of varied temperaments. The faith-oriented person, the person for whom trust, selflessness, surrender and a prayerful attitude come easily, can practice the path of prayer—Bhakti Yoga. The will and reason-oriented can practice Hatha, Karma, Kriya and Raja Yogas with equally effective results.

Eventually all paths of yoga—both the path of prayer and the path of will—are designed to awaken the dormant energy know as Kundalini Shakti. As the active Shakti begins to automatically hasten the practitioner's growth, he naturally enters the path of surrender, in which devotion and faith play a predominant role. When the follower of the path of will reaches this stage, however, he experiences faith naturally as a result of his concrete experience of growth in the earlier stage of practice. Faith is not demanded at the outset of the search. Instead it develops gradually and naturally as a result of sustained, willful practice.

Whether God comes from above or exists within makes no difference to those who have experienced the heights of higher consciousness, but it does make a difference to beginners. Sometimes a misunderstanding as to the most suitable path for an individual may retard the growth of even the most sincere seeker. The path that begins from man, from the known, is naturally much easier for most people to follow. The path of will and action is readily understood and practiced by most Westerners, who have habitually relied upon logic and reason. Total surrender and faith are very hard to come by in this age of reason and science.

The path of prayer—the path of surrender—is a difficult path for most beginners. The beauty of yoga lies in the fact that each individual can follow the path most suited to his nature, for yoga teaches that all paths lead to the same place—to the divine within.

# Prana and Its Mysteries Unveiled

The all-pervading cosmic energy is known as prana. Prana is nature's secret key. It is the basic unit, the primal energy from which all creation has emerged. One who knows the mysteries of prana can unlock the secrets of the self and the universe, for the entire universe is an expression of prana. Even though different trees and plants may derive their nutrition from the same earth, the same water, the same sun and air, they manifest a wide variety of fruits, flowers, leaves, colors, shapes and sizes. In the same way, prana, although it is one energy, multiplies itself and manifests through a variety of names and forms. Stars, moon, planets, sun, earth, vegetable life and animal life—all are the expressions of prana.

In its early, evolutionary stages, prana formed the five elements of earth, water, fire, air and ether, out of which emerged the entire vegetable and animal kingdoms. It was the pranic life force which generated the evolution of these kingdoms. After millions of years, at the peak of these evolutionary processes, man stands as the pinnacle of pranic manifestation.

In yogic scriptures, prana is described as the residual power of Brahman, the cosmic being, the creative force in the universe. Brahman is the ultimate source from whom all has emerged and into whom all will eventually merge. Brahman is the source, the unmanifest, and prana is his expression, his extension, his manifestation. Brahman is the source of creation and prana is the energy which assumes a variety of forms to become creation itself. Brahman represents the male principle, and pranic energy, the female principle or mother nature. This duality is described symbolically in Hindu mythology as Krishna and Radha or Shiva and Shakti.

The process of the creative source and its creation through prana takes place within each individual. When a child is conceived, the brain is formed first, followed by the spinal cord, which is in turn followed by the formation of the rest of the body. The life, the prana, enters the fetus through the fontanelle, the very soft and pulsating place on the top of the head of a newly born baby. After entering the body through the top of the head, this divine universal energy spreads to the nervous system of the spine to form the rest of the body. Just as the entire universe is composed of prana assuming various forms, so the varied parts of the human body are all the expressions of pranic energy, the creative force in man. Completing its task, prana settles at the base of the spine, resting in the pelvic coccygeal plexus known in yoga as Muladhara Chakra. In this state, prana assumes the form known to yogis as the sleeping Kundalini Shakti, man's dormant evolutionary energy.

The top of the head is the seventh and highest chakra (nerve plexus), the abode and seat of the causal cosmic being, symbolically named Brahman, Shiva, Krishna, or in the West, God the Father. In the **Bhagavad Gita**, this phenomenon is described as the tree of life whose roots extend above while its branches extend below (Chapter 15:1). This tree of life represents the nervous and glandular systems. The brain is the root of life energy, the spinal column, the main passageway for the energy. The spinal column is like the trunk of the tree with the nerves as branches. In the spinal column exist the six plexus (known as chakras) which eventually connect to the source, the brain, the Brahman, and also to the pituitary and pineal glands, both of which are housed in the highly-protected chamber of the skull. The highest chakra is symbolically described as a lotus with a thousand petals while the other chakras, or lotuses, in the spine have been described as having fewer number of petals. The canal through which the energy travels, the passage of the nervous system, is called the Shushumna, which extends from the base of the spinal cord to the cerebral center, connecting the first chakra, the Muladhara, to the seventh and highest chakra, the Sahasrara.

For the first seven years of life, and in some cases

longer, the Shushumna is open. The pranic energy flows freely between the Muladhara and Sahasrara (although this age of purity is decreasing as the race "advances"). As a result, the child enjoys union with Brahman. He enjoys freedom from past and future, freedom from fear and desires, freedom from selfishness and ego. In short, he possesses all the qualities of a most highly-developed and evolved Siddha (master), enjoying total communion with God. This is why Christ says, "Unless you change and become like little children, you will never enter the Kingdom of Heaven." (Matthew 18:3).

We cannot call a child enlightened, however, because the child has not yet transcended his ego. He carries, in dormant form, potential karma, the residual habit and thought patterns of previous lifetimes. As soon as his instrument of the body becomes mature enough to handle his potential karma, his ego becomes active. Now his karma begins to express itself as the ego-oriented tendencies and habits of the past come to life again. Although the child appears to be pure until this point, he is not pure in actuality. He still has potential karma. He must experience the evolution of this karma with its accompanying desires, hopes, habit patterns, expectations and aspirations. Christ does not say that if you are a child you will enter the kingdom of heaven. Instead he says that you must become like a child. He implies a process of becoming child-like, of becoming pure, spontaneous and living in the present moment. He implies that man must become child-like by consciously transcending the traps of the ego, by growing through the stage of infancy and by consciously overcoming the past-earned karmic patterns to enter the state of communion with God. At the completion of this process, what remains is man's true nature, Sat-Chit-Ananda (Truth-Consciousness-Bliss). This is the meaning of the Biblical teaching that man is made in the image and likeness of God. As one cuts through the clouds of ignorance and selfishness, the light, the love, the purity and the glory of the Father already dormant in man begins to shine through more and more.

A child's ego is dormant. It awaits expression, which happens when the notion of separation—the notion of "I and mine", "you and me"—enters his consciousness. This phenomenon is very much like that of a patient in a coma who has a dormant pain potential. In the unconscious state, he does not seem to suffer, but as soon as he becomes conscious, the dormant pain and suffering return. So also as the child becomes conscious on an ego level of a separate identity, he begins to lose the God-like purity, the love and the bliss.

Here we can clearly see the secret behind man's separation from his true nature, from his Father. As long as the child is one with the Father in the highest chakra and lives in total harmony with nature, the child is taken care of by the divine Father within him. As soon as the ego separates him from the Father, however, the fear of the "other" begins. The ego brings the "other" into existence. The stronger the ego, the greater is the distance between man and God, between man and the "other". The stronger the ego, the greater is the threat and fear of the "other".

This concept is explained allegorically in the story of Adam and Eve. As long as Adam was in total union with the Creator, as long as he was united with Brahman in the highest chakra, there was no shame, no desire, no dualism. There was no "other". He was in the consciousness of "My Father, Thy will be done, not mine." He lived in the total union and experience of "I am in the Father and the Father is in me." (John 14:11). As soon as the individual ego desired, he separated from the Father. This separation is the growth of the ego. From this point on, Adam becomes the prodigal son who separates from his true home and oneness with his Father in the seventh chakra, the thousand-petalled lotus. He separates from his true nature of bliss and paradoxically goes out in search of bliss on his own, through his individual ego. His consciousness starts on a journey, descending to progressively lower and lower states. From Sahasrara Chakra, he descends through each successively lower chakra until he settles at the lowest level of consciousness, the Muladhara Chakra, at the base of the spine.

Each human being experiences the state of Adam and Eve. The child in the early stages of growth lives in the purity of Eden. He has no shame, no guilt. When his body becomes mature enough to handle his past-earned karma, however, this karma leads him into separation from the Father. He becomes conscious of the "other".

It is at this point that he encounters the serpent. The serpent who tempts Adam is man's ego, his desire for ego-centered gratification through the medium of sensual pleasure. Also representative of the Kundalini energy, the serpent symbolizes the life force in man which can either be dissipated through excessive sensual indulgence or conserved and transformed for inner growth. Sex is the most powerful desire because it is not merely a desire of the senses, but a desire for individual ego-oriented expression. It represents the ultimate desire of man to achieve bliss on his own, to experience the bliss of external union as opposed to the bliss provided by union with the Father inside himself. And so the snake, the sensual energy, the "id" described by Freud, makes his entry into man's consciousness, not so much as the desire for sex, but as the desire for ego expression. When man chooses the snake, when he decides to externalize his energies, he separates from the Father. Now he experiences shame and guilt because he is conscious of the "other".

The story of Adam and his temptation by the serpent is the story of man. Each person is an Adam. Each soul goes through the process of ego development, progressively getting caught deeper and deeper in the self-created cobweb of separation from the Father and alliance with the individual ego identity. This process is the story of the prodigal son. Man is this prodigal son who has come to rest in the lowest possible state of consciousness, dying of spiritual hunger, starving for energy "in a foreign land".

Just as each individual passes through these stages of consciousness in one lifetime, so also does mankind in general. The levels of conciousness of the human race are described in the ancient yogic scriptures as yugas (ages)— Satya Yuga, Dwapara Yuga, Treta Yuga and Kali Yuga. Each age marked a stage of consciousness of mankind in general.

In Satya Yuga, man was in his pure conscious state. He lived a life of Ajna Chakra, the center of intuitive wisdom, the meeting point of consciousness and superconsciousness. In Dwapara Yuga, he lives a life of Vishuddha Chakra, the center of intuitive spontaneity. In Treta Yuga, he lives a life of Anahata Chakra, the center of compassion, and, in the darkest ages of Kali Yuga, man lives a life of the three lowest chakras, the Manipura, Swadhisthana and Muladhara. Each of these lower centers represents externalized, ego-centered, power and lust-oriented energy. Thus man progressively lowered his consciousness until he descended into the darkest age, in which the prana of the average person was active mainly in the three lower chakras. The divine consciousness sleeps at the base of the spine. It cannot go any lower. Now the ascending cycle of ages has begun again. At the threshold of Dwapara Yuga, man begins to lift his consciousness to its original state of oneness in the highest chakra.

On his return journey to the highest man must pass successively through each state of consciousness he once passed on his journey away from the Father. On the path of Kundalini Yoga, this journey is made by the divine Kundalini energy which is aroused from its slumber in the Muladhara, the lowest chakra and raised to the Sahasrara, the highest chakra and the seat of cosmic consciousness. As the energy is raised, man passes through, experiences and finally transcends each level of consciousness inherent in each chakra.

This process is a slow and evolutionary one. The aspirant must progress on the path with great patience, understanding and self-acceptance in order to transcend the

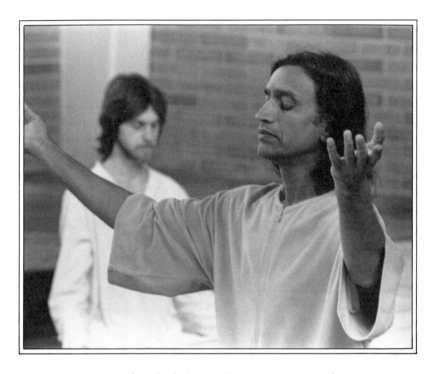

ego-trappings of each chakra and gain passage to the next chakra or level of consciousness. Although such evolutionary processes are very slow, they can be accelerated by awakening the energy of Kundalini Shakti through the practice of Kundalini Yoga. Once activated, the Shakti speeds up this process, helping man raise his consciousness to higher and higher levels within a very short time. What otherwise could take lifetimes to accomplish can be accomplished within a very short period through the potent power of Kundalini Shakti.

When an individual's prana expresses itself primarily through the first chakra, he lives his life in a state of sleep and ignorance. Such a person's primary drive is the search for security. He acts out his stereotyped, everyday routine with the goal of being safe, being protected, being secure. First chakra man has learned to see himself only in terms of security and survival. He lives with security as his primary motive, hiding himself behind his basic security demands.

108     Although externally he may appear to be content with his dream world, he is actually driven by fears, deep tensions and the constant need to insure his own survival by acquiring food, possessions, and the articles that provide his imagined security. He is not motivated to overcome these fears nor does he see any way to overcome them. He is unwilling to direct his effort towards any goal but further security. He is lazy and asleep.

Second chakra man has been roused from the lethargy of dullness and insensitivity experienced in the first chakra. When prana is expressed through the second chakra, man begins to explore the sensual pleasures of the external world. He views others as potential instruments for the satisfaction of his desires. He searches constantly for that which will fulfill his desires, trying every available material method to meet his sensual wants. This person becomes totally dependent on the outside world for his happiness. When his desires are temporarily met, he experiences great bursts of excitement. When the object of his desire is withdrawn, he becomes the victim of deep depressions and internal emptiness.

When prana enters the realm of the third chakra, the drive for power becomes man's primary motivation. He searches for prestige, respect, admiration and wealth. Third chakra man becomes adept at manipulating—he manipulates his friends, his co-workers, his family, his wife— all are sacrificed to his relentless need for power. Such a man lives in a state of constant fear. Until he reaches his goal, he fears failure. When he reaches it, when he gains power, he fears the loss of it. No matter how successful he becomes in his search, at the end of each victory still greater possibilities and desires lure him on. He can never be satisfied, because all his power desires are imaginary ones. Every time he successfully achieves his goal, his imagination creates new desires. He can never enjoy the fruits of his success.

Although the three lower chakras represent security,

passion and power, they are not considered to be bad. Chakras are doors through which energy is expressed. They are simply aspects of man's nature, functions which may be used for higher or lower purposes. The energy of sex, for example, is a divine energy. When used only for sensual gratification, however, it becomes a great source of unhappiness in man's life. Yoga does not condemn the lower chakras; yoga teaches man to transcend them. The wise use of the energy expressed through the lower chakras leads man to higher and higher states of consciousness. The same energies which can bind man to a life of tension, aggression, fear and depression can, when properly channeled through yogic methods, become the very vehicles for his ascent to superconsciousness.

The spiritual path begins with the fourth chakra. When prana radiates from the heart chakra, it is mobilized by compassion. Love is the source of energy for an individual acting from this center. Such a person lives in the world but beyond it, like the lotus flower which grows in the water and yet remains untouched by the water. He is in the process of transcending the demands of ego. He is beginning to rise above his selfishness, seeing the world with the eye of compassion, love and universal brotherhood. Such a man is learning to go beyond the pains, miseries and fears to which the lower chakra person is prone. He has realized that the kingdom of heaven is within—he has begun his spiritual journey.

Yoga means union. It systematically teaches man to raise his energies to ever higher and more subtle levels of expression in order to experience the state of inner union. Once these energies are transformed to higher levels, there is little energy remaining for use in lower forms of expression. Gone is the compulsion to compete, compare or to indulge in self-destructive gratification. In the place of compulsion comes freedom—the freedom that allows man a continued state of evolvement, a progressive unfolding of his longed-for union with the Father who is his true self.

# The Chakras

| Chakra | Location | Corresponding Physical Nerve Plexus | Corresponding Physical Gland | Corresponding Physical Sense Organ |
|---|---|---|---|---|
| Sahasrara | crown of the head | pineal gland | pineal gland | consciousness (chitta) |
| Ajna | space between the eyebrows | cavernous plexus | pituitary gland | intellect (buddhi) |
| Vishuddha | throat | laryngeal plexus | thyroid gland | ears |
| Anahata | heart | cardiac plexus | thymus gland | skin |
| Manipura | navel | solar plexus (epigastric plexus) | adrenal glands | eyes |
| Swadhisthana | reproductive organs | parastatic plexus | spleen | tongue |
| Muladhara | between the anus and reproductive organs | sacral plexus | gonads, ovaries | nose |

| Corresponding Organ of Action | Element | Function | Color | Number of Petals or Yogic Channels of Energy |
|---|---|---|---|---|
| beyond action | void— beyond elements | transcendent consciousness | luminosity | 1000 |
| mind | mind | dream consciousness | luminosity | 2 |
| legs | ether | heating | blue | 16 |
| palms and fingers | air | touch | smoke | 12 |
| feet | fire | sight | red | 10 |
| reproductive organs | water | taste | white | 6 |
| anus | earth | smell | yellow | 4 |

**Note:** Due to the nature of this work, a complete and highly technical depiction of the chakras, involving excessive Sanskrit terminology, is not given.

112       From the fourth to seventh chakras, the journey toward union begins. In these chakras, man reaches higher and higher states of consciousness, eventually breaking the tie of the ego and growing above all duality. He merges with superconsciousness, entering the state called Samadhi—complete and ultimate union with the Father.

## God Is Energy

All life is a play of energy. Man constantly searches for this energy in the sense that he constantly searches for peace, happiness, health, well-being, fulfillment, contentment and joy. When man lacks these qualities, he tries innumerable methods of gaining them. Such qualities, however, are no more than the by-products of energy.

Energy is strength; it is security. When man is high in energy, he commands great inner capacities. He holds the solution to all problems because his energy itself is the solution. When the same man becomes low in energy, however, he at once feels depressed, insecure, fearful. Problems overwhelm him and no solution seems to work. A host of enemies in the form of tensions, worries, aggressions, hatred, jealousy and competition appear to further deplete the little energy he has. His life is an energy crisis, a crisis full of doubts and questions which come as his energy is depleted. These doubts and questions are no more than reflections of man's basic lack of energy.

Man searches for energy in a variety of ways. He searches through his ego—through the desire for security, sensual stimulation or power. This search is a search within shadows—it is a never-ending effort to catch a phantom. The energy of the ego's shadow world is energy in name only. It has the external appearance of true energy, but lacks the true substance of the sustaining energy which man really seeks. Because this imitation energy is visible, tangible and easily accessible, however, the average man is willing to accept it. Such a man wants results quickly and so he is willing to settle for second best. Man can quickly command the energy of ego, but behind the immediate feeling of pleasure and security produced by such energy lies an army of disappointments, sorrow, suffering, pain, loneliness and fear. Hitler commanded very powerful energy, yet everywhere he went he created destruction, pain and suffering.

It is energy man wants, but he thinks he wants money; he thinks he wants possessions; he thinks he wants power. He really wants none of these things; all he really wants is energy. When man possesses energy, it becomes his security, it becomes his wealth, it becomes everything to him. The person who lacks energy tries to replace it in many different ways and still he remains unfulfilled.

The highest energy is love. The manifestation of love energy is peace, tranquility, contentment, joy, happiness and compassion. In order for the ego to be fulfilled, man channels his energy outwardly. Then the inner being suffers. To command the energy of love, he must conserve his energy and transform it into higher consciousness. Love energy does not generate as much external prosperity as does ego energy, but it gives far greater inner prosperity in the form of peace of mind, emotional and mental health and inner happiness. Paradoxically, these are the very qualities which man seeks through the self-defeating externalization of ego-generated energy.

Love is the highest energy. God is love. God is the highest source of energy which exists. There is no such thing as a disbeliever in God. Every man is searching for energy and God is energy. The energy that is God, however, cannot be studied and observed like the energy of electricity. God is a subtle energy, a force beyond the grasp of the mind and the senses. God is infinite, incomparable. His energy never began, nor will it ever end. God is the highest energy, the source of all energies. For this reason there is only one God. There is no parallel to Him, no

114      comparison to Him. He is without attributes.

Although God is beyond the mind, man has tried to comprehend God through his mind. Instead of realizing that he is made in the image and likeness of God, man has tried to create God in his own image and likeness. The result of man's efforts is not one, but many gods for man— all products of his own fantasies and imaginations. Man's image of God is the product of his mind and ego, a mind and ego which are incapable of ever truly comprehending God. The real perception of God is a transcendental experience—an experience which can only be reached in the higher dimensions of meditation. God cannot be comprehended or contained in the mind, because the mind itself is incomplete—it is only a part of the whole. God, the universal mind, is the whole. The part cannot contain the whole, it can only become one with the whole. Thus man's mind cannot contain God. The process of uniting with the whole is the process of knowing God. When a yogi reaches the highest state of consciousness, his individuality is removed and he becomes one with God.

Man tries to know God through his mind. He labels God as "good" or "bad", "merciful" or "condemning". God is neither good nor bad, neither merciful nor condemning. God is a neutral process of energy in movement, an energy which, like electricity, can be utilized by man in whatever way he chooses. When man attributes qualities to God, he tries to set comprehensible limits and boundaries on God's incomprehensible, limitless nature. What is good cannot be bad. God, however, is beyond such qualities. He is beyond boundaries.

Reality cannot be divided. God, the ultimate reality, is one. There is nothing that exists apart from him. For a boundary to exist it is necessary that there be the "other". Your house has boundaries only because there are other properties around it. The world has boundaries because it is surrounded by space. God is one. There is nothing that exists beyond him. Everything exists within him, for God is the energy which constitutes every object in the material and non-material worlds.

Man conceives of a God who sits up in heaven, rewarding the good and punishing the wicked. This is not the case. God has no favorites. He grants no concessions, no favors. When man asks God for favors, he makes a change within himself and believes that God has granted him the favor. When man prays, he answers his own prayers by his own effort, by his own ability to gain and sustain a high energy level.

Man believes that God answers his prayers, but in reality the answering of his prayers—the working of God within him—occurs through his own efforts and positive thought patterns. Every thought is a prayer to the God who is man's own inner energy. Positive thoughts create certain responses within the body, mind and emotions and thus generate positive results. In the same way, negative thoughts become a negative prayer. When man thinks self-destructive thoughts, he is stamping negative impressions upon his consciousness. These thoughts eventually actualize in the form of deep, self-destructive complexes. Thus man's prayers are always answered by the God within him.

Prayer is only a stage of going towards God. It is only one wing, while effort is the other. Without two wings the bird of divine grace cannot fly. Action in accordance with prayer is prayer solidified. If you pray but do not act accordingly, you are not truly praying. On the other hand, you may act according to your higher nature and never consciously pray, yet that act becomes a prayer in action, a prayer which is much more powerful than verbal prayer unaccompanied by action. A person may not even believe in God, but he can receive the grace of God by living a life harmonious with God's energy.

Prayer opens you to God. It removes the veils of ignorance by calling your attention to God. God's grace is like the sunshine. When there are clouds between you and the sun, you cannot feel the sun's warmth, but when the clouds are removed, you receive its grace, its warming energy. The

116 sun is always shimmering and shining. In the same manner, God continually showers His grace. You need only remove the barriers which separate you from God's energy to experience His grace.

To say that God either gives to you or takes away from you is a misconception. God treats all equally. He does not give mercy, but when you go closer to God, you are more able to feel His mercy. God showers His mercy in the same way a flower showers its fragrance. The flower continually gives forth its fragrance, but you must draw close in order to appreciate it. The closer you come to the energy of God the more bliss and happiness you experience. The farther away you move, the lower will be your energy, the more pain, suffering, alienation, loneliness, fear and frustration you will experience. When man receives God's grace, it is a result of man's living closer to God's laws, the laws of nature, the laws of energy. When a man lives in harmony with these laws, he feels happy and content. Then man says he lives with God's grace. These results do not come about because God favors him, however, but because he is living in harmony with the laws of God. When man no longer follows these laws, he moves away from God. That does not mean that God is judging him, but that he is separating himself from God by going against the laws of nature, the universal laws of energy. Then he suffers and blames God for being so ruthless, so merciless. Actually man's suffering is the result of his own choice. There is no such thing as a God of grace or a God of judgement. Grace and judgement are the result of man's own action, his own doing. God's grace is always available. Man decides whether to receive that grace by moving closer to God or farther away from Him.

Man is made in the image and likeness of God, who is energy itself. When he allows his energy to become low — when he draws away from God, he no longer experiences his true nature. He no longer experiences God.

God neither forgives nor punishes, but He does give the continual opportunity to grow closer to Him. Every moment is an opportunity to make a transition, a transformation in man's life. Man has the choice to allow his energy to rise high and become God-like or to dissipate his energy through wrong thinking and living habits. Because God is always the same, the laws of the universe are always uniform; they are never changing. They are constant and equal in their action and reaction. These laws are God in action. If God could change, then the laws of the universe could change. Can you imagine the laws of electricity and gravity working one day, but not the next?

God is everywhere and in everyone. He is in everything animate and inanimate. He is everywhere and He is nowhere. Because He has no shape, He can take on all shapes; because He has no attributes, He can take on all attributes. God is indefinable—beyond definition. He is beyond form, and so He takes on all forms.

God is simply an energy. He doesn't "know" in the way that we know with the mind. The mind knows only in terms of good and bad, but God does not know in that sense. Yet He knows all. His "knowing" is like the "knowing" of electricity. Electricity does not know a good man from a bad man—whoever touches it receives a shock. To know the laws of God is man's responsibility. If he ignores these laws he suffers, just as if he ignores electricity he will receive a shock or if he ignores fire he will get burned. Only if he knows the laws of nature will he be able to use nature for his own benefit. Then he can say God is favoring him. It is not God's grace which favors him, however, but the knowledge which gives him the ability to use God's laws for his comfort, happiness and growth. That is how knowledge makes man free. The knowledge of God is not only the knowledge of the material world, but also knowledge of God's internal laws. When all of God's laws are understood, all inhibitions are released and all energy becomes totally one—totally in harmony with the universal energy. Then man transcends his nature and becomes one with God, one with existence.

118    As an energy, God is everywhere. That means He
exists even in the devil. But because God is beyond the
attributes of good and evil, the duality of devil and divine
does not exist.

To live a life of attunement with God, you must live a
life that dissipates a minimum amount of energy. Total
union with God means losing no energy. Then you and
energy become one. You and God become one.

The yogi who reaches a high level of consciousness
seems to defy the laws of the universe, but he does not. He
merely has achieved a deeper understanding, a mastery of
the universal laws. The path of yoga leads you to union
with God by teaching you how to understand the laws of
God, the laws of the universal energy. Once you understand that God is without attribute, you stop blaming God
for your happiness or unhappiness. Then you begin to
change yourself. It is these inner changes which allow you
to grow close to God by being open to His energy.

The higher states of consciousness cannot be achieved
through mental comprehension. God cannot be comprehended, but He can be experienced. To penetrate the infinite nature of God, you must transcend your finite nature
by sacrificing your desires. Those qualities which result
from desire, such as lust, greed, selfishness and hatred pull
you away from God because they deplete your energy.

You may contemplate God on a personal level as a
being within your heart, or you may see Him on an imper-
sonal level as an energy. The approach does not matter.
What is important is that you remove the barriers which
create disharmony between you and the universe—which
separate you from your divine self. When you are separated
from God's energy, you feel alienated and fearful. There is
no harmony in the world for you. When you contact that
source of energy which is God, however, happiness and
harmony become a part of your nature.

Because God exists within everything, He exists within
man himself. In man, God is expressed as life energy—the

process of creation, sustenance, dissolution and evolution occurring continually within man's body. In the **Bhagavad Gita** (an ancient yogic scripture), it is said, "I become the digestive fire and digest the food." Yogis believe that all bodily processes—respiration, digestion, circulation, metabolism, elimination—are the workings of God Himself. All processes are sustained and controlled through the inner energy which is God within man.

The ancient yogic texts allude to God residing within man by describing actual "deities" which are believed to dwell in the various nerve centers of man's body. These "deities" are the specific forms of subtle energy which exist within the nervous system. Through the practice of Mantra Yoga, potent sound formulas corresponding to the various "deities" are chanted to purify the subtle nerves of each center, to refine their functions and to remove blockages which prevent man's energy from rising to higher levels. Thus the "deities" described in yoga are neither abstract concepts nor imaginary divine personages—they are the most intimate energies of life itself.

Because God exists in man, man must honor his body and its processes to truly honor God. When man hurts, blocks, pollutes or distorts the rhythm of nature, either within or outside himself, he is hurting God. Harmony with God is harmony with the internal and external world—harmony which begins in man as a balance of body, mind and emotions. When this harmony exists, God is "pleased". In other words, man experiences a balanced flow of his inner energies with his environment, a flow which is expressed as physical health, emotional maturity and mental tranquility. This tranquility is none other than "the peace that passeth all understanding", a peace which does not arise from the mind, but from the direct experience of oneness with God.

Because God lives in man, what is known as "sin" is any act which obstructs or disturbs the harmonious flow of energies within man himself. Any act described as "sin" by

120     any great religion has a disturbing effect upon the individual on either a physical, mental, emotional or spiritual level. Such acts deplete man of his vital energies; they rob him of health and destroy his peace of mind. For this reason, they are acts "against" God—acts which disrupt man's inner and outer rhythm of energies.

Yoga provides practical methods to remedy the "sins" of inner disturbance which obstruct man's oneness with God. Each method available in yoga is precisely designed to maximize inner harmony, lead to a balanced flow of life energies for total physical, mental, emotional and spiritual well-being. In so doing, they allow man to transcend his body, mind and ego. This transcendence eventually leads him to oneness with the infinite ocean of energy called God.

Although each of the many approaches of yoga lead man to greater harmony with the divine energy inside his body, it is through Shaktipat Kundalini Yoga that man experiences the most profound working of this energy. On this path, the dormant but potent inner energy known as Kundalini Shakti is awakened from its sleep at the base of man's spine. Thus Shakti is the individualized essence of God Himself, the creative and evolutionary force innate but inactive in each man. Through Shaktipat (psychic transferral of energy), the deserving aspirant receives the spark of spiritual awakening from a Guru (spiritual teacher). With this transferral, the universal energy of Shakti awakens inside the recipient's body. Acting through its own universal intelligence, this power of God within undertakes the automatic work of cleansing the body, mind and emotions. Energies which have long been trapped in frozen and tense muscles, nerves and glands are released along with their corresponding psychological and emotional blockages. The awakened Shakti works through the nervous and endocrine systems, purifying the physical and subtle nerves in a very precise, scientific manner, specifically designed to meet the individual's immediate needs and temperament. Through this process, the awakened Shakti

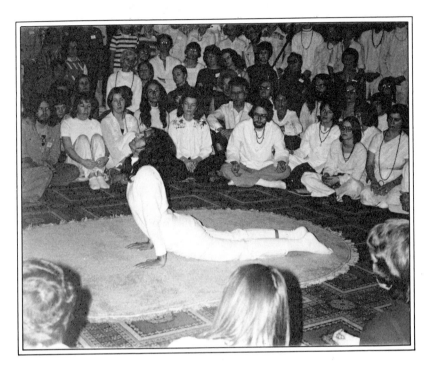

removes all forms of disease at their roots. It tones, purifies and harmonizes the entire nervous and glandular systems and restores the body to its true and forgotten role as the temple of God.

The awakened Shakti accomplishes its preliminary purification and strengthening of the body, particularly the nervous system, so that the potent energy of God can work through the strong, steel-like nerves of the yogi and lead him to superconscious states. Those who lack contact with a Master capable of imparting Shakti can, however, accomplish this preparatory purification through the willful practice of Yama and Niyama, along with Hatha, Karma and Mantra Yogas. These willful practices are very time-consuming and can become dry and tedious even under the guidance of an expert teacher. Eventually these conscious practices, if done with dedication and perseverance, can also awaken the Kundalini energy. The significance of Shaktipat, however, lies in the fact that the process is automatic. It is accomplished from within, through the all-knowing power of God called prana. In willful practice, man must consciously decide which methods best suit his needs. There exists the problem of making wrong decisions, based on an intellectual misunderstanding of available information. Shakti eliminates this problem, because it works automatically through its own intelligence. All methods emerge spontaneously from within, in direct and natural response to man's deepest inner needs.

Through Shaktipat, the disciple receives an immediate and continued experience of God's energy within. Such an experience makes God understandable on a practical level. It enables the disciple to grow beyond his energy-draining defenses to experience the bliss and happiness that God's energy gives. In this way, the disciple develops his own God-like, super-human qualities through the accelerated evolutionary processes set in motion by Kundalini. God is not a mental conception, but a transcendental experience. Through the path of Shaktipat Kundalini Yoga, the individual gains access to this direct experience.

## Melting into Oneness

Man craves union with God. He seeks oneness with the divine force which exists within him as energy. In the purity of childhood, man experienced oneness. He now longs to recapture the bliss of inner union lost beneath the demands of his adult ego. He longs to forget the self—the small self, the fearful self, the conscious self—and merge into union with his source. Despite this longing, however, he has activated his mind and ego to such an extent that he is no longer able to experience such oneness. He has activated his mental faculties to such a degree that, even when he enters an area of life where the mind is not necessary, he persists on using the mind. At night, for example, the mind should be set aside for a restful, deep sleep. Many people, however, have such excessively active minds that they cannot do this, at least not without drugs.

Man has not learned how to shut down the mind. That is why so many people have difficulty experiencing a sexual orgasm. The joy of climax, depends entirely on transcending the mind and ego. The one condition of experiencing the bliss of sex is to completely lose identification with the body, mind and social identity, and to become entirely at one with the flow of energy. The average man with a highly charged mind and ego cannot do this. He has abused his mind so much, exaggerating its importance so far out of proportion to its real function, that he now tries to let it take over all bodily functions. In the sex act, for example, the entire body must participate in the experience. Because man has not learned to do this, he makes a futile attempt at accomplishing the work of the sex center with the mind and thus enters the world of sexual fantasy, even during the sex act itself. This mental process is self-defeating, for it will never take man into the true experience of union.

The mind is the obstruction—the veil. It is constantly expecting, demanding, comparing, contesting, craving, complaining, projecting, interpreting and evaluating. All these functions require and expend a great deal of energy. The mind feeds on energy. It uses and misuses energy to fulfill its functions, to complete its mental processes—and to assure its own survival. When the mind is temporarily suspended, the energy it normally consumes is released to flow to the rest of the body. The ultimate experience of such a state of mental suspension is the yogic state of Samadhi. In Samadhi, every gland, each and every cell, the entire chemistry of the body, responds to the merging—to the mystery of melting into oneness with God. The entire flow of energy vibrates and rushes in rhythm and harmony with existence. The entangled, strangled consciousness of the mind becomes free to soar high and unite with the supreme consciousness—the cosmic consciousness known as God. This is the final state of oneness which man instinc-

124    tively and unconsciously craves.

While man craves ultimate union, however, he also fears it. It is a threat to him, for the unknown is always threatening. Man is afraid to let go of the solid ground of the known and jump into the depths of the ocean of the unknown. He is afraid to lose himself—to lose his identity, his ego. He wants to feel secure, no matter what the cost. For this reason, he strives to make everything known.

Man has devised many ways out of this predicament of wanting the oneness experience and yet fearing it. He has resorted to external methods of stimulating his nervous system in an attempt to capture the ecstasy of union—the unknown—while remaining within the realm of the known. These methods create substitute experiences which resemble the original, real experience of oneness by creating temporary spans of mental suspension. Whenever the mind is transcended or suspended, even momentarily, an explosion of ecstasy is the result.

Man is in a constant, unending search of these explosions of energy. Many of his most popular pastimes have been devised just to produce such rushes of ecstasy. Horror movies create such experiences. The suspense draws the viewer in through his identification with the "hero". In the moment of peak suspense and horror, the mind is suspended—it goes into a swoon. If the identification is strong, the viewer goes into states of consciousness similar to those portrayed by the hero with whom he identifies. His experience is comparable to that of the hero. If the identication is weak, the experience will be less intense, for it is through identification that energy is contacted. When a child watches a horror movie or reads a suspense story, his identication is very intense. He becomes completely absorbed in the drama of the story. The adult, on the other hand, knows that it is an imaginary story, that "it is not really happening". For this reason, his experience is less intense than that of the child.

Dangerous sports and adventures such as car and mo-

torcycle racing, bullfighting, mountain climbing, or cross-
ing the Atlantic in a hand-made boat, are other examples of
man's search for ecstasy. These adventures take man into
life or death situations. They challenge life. At such critical
times, the average mind is incapable of coping with the
magnitude of the problem. The urgency of the situation
automatically alerts the entire human mechanism to penetrate the higher dimensions of superconsciousness in order
to cope with the existing emergency—and hence the ecstasy, the climax, the transcendence into the region of no
thought, of pure consciousness.

The possibility of deriving ecstasy from such situations is directly proportional to the degree of risk involved.
The greater the chance of death (or, in the case of today's
materialistic society, the more fantastic the monetary reward for success), the greater is man's absorption. Absorption commands a tremendous amount of energy. When
man craves such energy and yet lacks the capacity or brav-
ery to face an authentic life or death situation, he resorts to
second-hand ecstasy by watching others engaged in life or
death struggles. The great popularity of dangerous or bru-
tal spectator sports, as well as the widespread appeal of
books and movies about war and violence, illustrates man's
craving for vicarious fear, excitement and absorption.

Man has devised many escapes, many substitute experiences to provide excitement in his life. Business adventures, gambling, excessive sex, the use of drugs and alcohol,
vandalism and other types of violence are just a few. The
basic factor in all such artificially created excitement is an
absorbing, all-consuming experience in which the mind is
put to sleep, enters a swoon state or becomes suspended
temporarily through fear, horror, suspense or excitement.
The goal behind each one of these experiences is instant
ecstasy. Not only does man want ecstasy, he wants it now.
He wants oneness quickly and easily. He is not willing to
put any effort into a sustained search, a true inquiry.

The main drawback of all these substitute experiences

126 is that, even though they may create temporary suspensions of the mind, they also carry with them many harmful side effects. No sooner are they finished than they bring tension and fear directly proportional to the degree of restlessness and insecurity which originally created them. They are temporary in nature and thus they require repetition. The repetition itself causes the effects of the act to deteriorate with time, as the nerves become immune to old, external stimuli. The very act which once gave bliss and joy eventually becomes tedious, boring and mechanical. By now, however, the self-created need for external excitation of the nerves has created a restless, relentless craving which progressively deprives man of his capacity to enjoy the act. The endless craving leads to frustration, which in turn leads to greater dependence on bigger and better stimulants resulting in greater insecurity, fear, anger and sorrow. Sensitivity and receptivity are reduced, and dullness, laziness, lethargy and insensitivity are induced. The act has now become a habit.

Seen at its greatest depth, each of these artificial methods is a means of searching for God; yet all such forms of man-made suspense and excitement are avoidances—avoidances of the search within. Man's true nature is Sat-Chit-Ananda (Truth-Consciousness-Bliss). It is every man's deepest, but often unconscious desire to return to his true nature. This return begins within—with knowing the body, the mind and the emotions, with seeing, understanding and working on the real issues that lead to permanent solutions of all man's problems. All artificially created experiences of oneness are man's attempts at forgetting himself by drowning his separateness, his pain at being alone. They become self-created traps, for they keep man so engaged in the vicious and self-defeating cycle of dependence on artificial excitement that he can afford to avoid the true search of life, the search for the Self.

The search for the Self is the search for God, for God is not separate from man. He dwells within man and works through him. Artificially created methods of transcending the mind are not part of this search. They are, in fact, detrimental to it. Methods of transcending the mind which can help man in his search are called meditation techniques. These methods gradually and naturally lead man to a conscious and controlled suspension of the mind. When the mind is suspended through natural means, i.e. through meditation techniques for the purpose of spiritual growth, an expansion of consciousness is the result. Man's life is transformed, and the inner union which he really seeks becomes a reality for him. When the mind is suspended through fear or suspense for the purpose of thrills, excitement, escape or ego gratification, there is no resulting positive change in man's life. Any apparent sense of oneness achieved through such methods is delusive and temporary, ultimately producing deeper states of dependence, depression and restlessness. Such externally-originated methods, even if they temporarily produce ecstasy and superior achievements, are artificial methods of expanding consciousness. Their results are temporary and destructive in nature.

Meditation is a natural method of expanding man's consciousness. It is a process that leads man step-by-step to self-realization, to the actualization of his inner, dormant potentials. It is the key to unlock the closed doors to the inner self, to the inner sanctuary of the Kingdom of Heaven within.

Meditation is losing the identity; it is becoming one with the infinite. It takes man beyond the mind, beyond time, beyond space—beyond the self-centered world of ego gratification. It is one method which gives man the true experience of union with God and opens him to the deepest and richest joys of life. These experiences are so profound that they make a permanent stamp of transformation on man's personality.

## The Slow Motion Prana Exercise:
### Experiencing Pranic Energy Through Deep Concentration

The pranic energy of God within can actually be experienced through a little known but powerful yogic technique. Through this technique, prana, which is generally controlled by the tyranny of the conscious mind, is released to move freely throughout the system. Once active, this inner intelligence purifies the body, recharging the entire system in a most effective manner. Through the Slow Motion Prana Exercise, the individual conscious will is temporarily surrendered to the universal will—to the inner guidance of pranic energy. As prana works throughout the system, it naturally restores the individual to a state of harmony and rhythm with the entire universe. Ordinarily man's mind distorts his natural functions and blocks the expression of his inner energies. The primary condition for practicing this method is to let go of the mind and temporarily surrender to the inner energy, which constantly seeks to restore balance between the individual and the universe. During the practice of this exercise, you simply let the energy of God within you take over.

This exercise was given to me personally by my beloved Gurudev, Swami Shri Kripalvanandji, a realized Master who has reached the highest state of God-realization, Nirvakalpa Samadhi. In the tradition of the great yogic teachings, this method stems from his direct personal experience. Realizing the nature of my mission in the West, Gurudev instructed me in this ancient and secret technique, saying "Teach this to your American students. This technique will be most successful and effective, winning the great admiration of its practitioner." With the blessings of so great a Master, I have taught this technique to thousands in the West for the past ten years. The benefits received by my students have been profound, transforming their lives on deep levels.

## How to Do the Exercise

This exercise is simple, but must be performed in extremely slow motion, accompanied by deep concentration on the flow of prana to certain areas of the body. The nature of the exercise is highly subtle, requiring deep attention to the inner movement of life energies.

Begin by sitting in the lotus pose or in a simple, cross-legged position. Keep your spine straight and hold your neck and back in alignment. Close your eyes and relax your body. Then begin to take long, deep and uniform breaths (perform Yogic Breathing if you are familiar with it). This deep breathing brings inner harmony, relaxes the body and calms the mind.

After several minutes of breathing, focus your attention upon the solar plexus, the storage battery of prana within the body. Imagine that the pranic energy is glowing in the solar plexus in the form of luminous, liquid light. Gradually visualize this prana streaming upward from the solar plexus and flowing gently through your arms, wrists, palms and into your fingers. Your fingertips may begin to vibrate with the great intensity of prana.

Continue concentrating on this energy flowing into your hands until you feel them being moved. Do not expect anything to happen. The key to this exercise is to concentrate on the prana and observe its working. Let your hands move toward your face in an extremely slow, almost invisible movement. If you feel that your hands are being moved without your conscious will, do not become alarmed. You are experiencing the workings of pranic energy. As your hands approach your face, allow your fingers to move gently across your face according to the patterns which arise spontaneously from within. As the fingertips move across the face, they discharge prana, relaxing deep muscles and erasing all lines.

Now allow your hands to return to their original position in the same slow, almost invisible motion. When they have come to rest, remain in a sitting position with your eyes closed for as long as you wish, staying attuned to the energy flowing within you.

### Student Reactions

The following comments were made by students after both observing and practicing the Slow Motion Prana Exercise.

"When I first saw Yogi Desai demonstrate the exercise, I felt very peaceful. I was amazed at the slowness. The first time I tried myself, it was jerky and by my own power, causing my shoulders to ache. More recently, it has given me daily rewards of rich meditation."

"During Yogi Desai's demonstration, I sensed a living power surging through his palms and fingertips and felt the overwhelming calm that permeated his being. When I tried the exercise myself, I felt that somehow my hands were being moved by something outside myself. The heaviness of my arms, plus the tingling sensation in my palms and fingertips made me realize that I too can benefit from this powerful flow of energy—prana."

"Watching Yogi Desai perform the exercise, I sensed his happiness, enjoyment, serenity and total involvement in what he was doing. He generated a certain peacefulness. When I reached the point in the technique where the palms were coming together, I was overcome by a strange, new pleasure. I stepped somewhere I had never been. My spirit seemed to transcend my body. I was totally aware of how I felt, yet somehow completely detached. I wanted to laugh, or was it cry?"

"At first I thought I must start moving my hands, but then I decided I would tell my hands to move themselves and then see if they would. I was amazed to see that they did. They were magnetically attracted to one another—gently, hesitantly, yet assuredly. So, I let my hands move. I

remember that each time I started thinking about something else (like 'I wonder if everyone else is going so slowly',
etc.), my hands stopped; so I tried concentrating on my
hands alone. This was an effort in the beginning, but it
came naturally after a while. It seemed like hours before my
hands met, but they finally did. When my hands touched,
my little trance was momentarily broken due to the shock
of the reality of my hands' flesh which until then seemed
numb and detached from my body. As I elevated my arms, I
was also quite aware and thinking—my arms didn't raise
themselves by themselves. I had to raise them. I was wide
awake and knew I was supposed to be thinking or feeling or
communicating about something, but I wasn't sure quite
what. Again I wondered what other people were thinking.
Also, my back started to hurt. In spite of all this, I felt
relaxed due to the tranquility in the room and the com-
mencing tranquility within myself. I felt much less self-
conscious than in the beginning when I had wondered what
I looked like. When I lowered my arms, a powerful force
overtook me and I felt drawn into a sort of heavy and calm
sleep. I tried to think but I couldn't. I tried to feel my body,
but I couldn't. My back no longer ached. Do you know how
it is when your leg has fallen asleep and then, when it
awakens, you have a sort of pricking feeling? Well, my
whole body felt like that. I just was. I don't remember
thinking anything at all. I do recall noticing that my hands
separated themselves automatically just as they had attracted themselves. I didn't really feel anything at the time.
Afterwards, I realized I must have been happy. I know I was
relaxed and had a hard time opening my eyes."

# Kundalini Yoga Through Shaktipat[1]

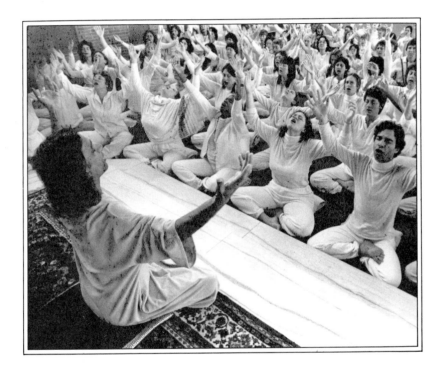

Kundalini Yoga is one of the most secret ancient sciences of India, but recently it has been made available to the West. Kundalini can be awakened by several different methods. There is Hatha Yoga—techniques of asana, pranayama, mudra and bandha (locks). There is Bhakti Yoga—the yoga of extreme love, devotion, faith, and mantra chanting. It can also be awakened suddenly and unex-

---

[1] Also appeared in: **Kundalini, Evolution and Enlightenment,** John White (ed.), (New York: Anchor, 1979).

134  pectedly as a result of incomplete sadhana (spiritual discipline) in a past life. In such cases, a person unfamiliar with the subject fails to understand the significance of the experience. If he is not actively searching for the results that this awakening ultimately brings, he will not benefit and progress. Some who experience this awakening without the guidance of a Guru become frightened, thinking it to be mental illness, nervousness, or evil spirits.

At such times the grace and guidance of an experienced Guru are necessary to sail safely through the varied experiences and attain samadhi (cosmic consciousness). Here it is necessary to point out that anyone who tries to awaken Kundalini through forced mechanical techniques without the guidance of an experienced master may encounter dangerous effects. Because Shaktipat is like a powerful charge, it is necessary that the nervous system be strong and pure.

## Guru's Grace

Many authors describe Kundalini Yoga as a dangerous approach. Yet the same could be said for learning to drive a car without the supervision of an expert driver. The safest and best method of awakening the Kundalini is through the grace of a realized Kundalini master. Even if Shakti is awakened by other means, the Guru's grace is essential on this path.

The Guru, when inspired by Divine Will, stirs up the latent Kundalini power in the deserving disciple. This process is called Shaktipat. The yogi who has control over prana can consciously bring his prana and his whole being to a certain level of vibration where he is able to impart it to others. The charismatic and magnetic influence of such masters can arouse the psychic astral force (Shakti) within the disciple. Swami Vishnu Tirtha, in his book *Devatma Shakti*, says, "Such great personalities have their prana and mind on higher potentiality and when approached they tend to raise the prana of others from a lower potentiality to a higher one."

A Guru transmits Shakti by a pregnant glance, touch, mantra, or simply by thought. Thus he installs his divine energy in his disciple, releasing mental and physiological blocks that had prevented the prana from moving freely within the body. The Guru, being in tune with his own master and with God, continues to receive Shakti uninterruptedly and abundantly in order to serve the spiritually hungry disciples. When Christians take Holy Communion, they are partaking of the flesh and blood of Christ. This was originally the act of receiving Christ's body into oneself. Similarly, with the Shaktipat initiation the disciple unites with his Guru and his love and faith increase as he progresses along the path.

Some receive Shaktipat by reading the writings of the master or by looking at his picture. This divine energy can be transferred at will or unconsciously. Simply touching any article which belongs to the Guru can ignite the spark within the disciple. Christ had this power. A woman who was ill came up behind him and touched his cloak. She was immediately healed, and Jesus, without seeing her, was aware of the occurrence. "Somebody hath touched me for I perceive that the power is gone out of me" (Luke 8:46).

## Shaktipat Diksha

During the process of Shaktipat Diksha (Shakti initiation), the astral body of the Guru merges with that of the disciple. It establishes karmic ties between the two which last for incarnations. At this time, the master takes on the karma of the initiate, thus speeding up the evolutionary process of his devotee. The same process of karmic ties is expressed in Christianity by the statement that Christ suffered and died for our sins (I Cor. 15:3). Not only did he take on the sins of men but he gave the power to disciples to do the same: "Receive ye the Holy Spirit: Whosoever sins ye remit, they are remitted unto them, and whosoever sins ye retain, they are retained" (John 20:23). The Shakti-

136   pat initiation creates an astral link between the Guru and disciple by which the disciple continues to receive psychic help from his chain of Gurus. Unity with the master is accomplished by complete surrender and love for the Guru accompanied by a special technique of meditation on the Guru (refer to *Play of Consciousness* by Swami Muktananda). The link which binds Guru and disciple in divine love grows, creating an almost irresistible pull on the aspirant to be near his master. Shaktipat opens an inner door which enables him to experience a tremendous amount of love. This is almost frightening to some who are not used to feeling such unconditional love. They temporarily suffer from typical Christian guilt feelings that they are unworthy of such blessings.

### How Shakti Works

Shaktipat Kundalini Yoga is the yoga of total surrender to God and Guru within. This is best accomplished by first surrendering to the external Guru and using him as a vantage point.

The phenomenon which occurs during and after Shaktipat initiation is the experience of surrender to the God-power (prana or Holy Spirit) within. It is this powerful divine force which becomes the inner protector and guide who is ever loving and forgiving once allowed to be free by the grace of the Guru. Through Shaktipat and an accompanying longing for freedom and knowledge on the part of the aspirant, the Shakti rises through the central canal of the spinal column (sushumna), piercing the six chakras (nerve plexuses). This is known as Kundalini awakening.

The aroused power of Kundalini affects both the autonomic nervous system, which functions by pranic intelligence alone, and the central nervous system, which functions under mental control. Under the effect of the powerful currents traveling through the entire nervous system as a result of Shaktipat, the prana assumes its original role as master of the whole being and the central nervous system becomes autonomic for a time. The mind under the influence of the boosted prana becomes a mute spectator of the divine inner intelligence. The prana becomes free from the usual mental tyrannies and functions as a purifying force wherever it is needed within the person. The *Atharva Veda*, one of the oldest Indian scriptures, says, ". . . bowing to the prana, under whose control is all this (universe), who is master of all, by whom everything is supported." So whenever the defenses of the mind are lifted and the prana level is raised, the prana's divine power accomplishes healing, purification and elevating effects in the body, mind, and spirit.

## Manifestations

When the empowered prana (Shakti) moves through the body, it creates various external and internal movements. On a physiological level one can experience the following: heat, cold, automatic breathing of various kinds, mudras, locks, postures (which are done with perfection even if the aspirant knows no Hatha Yoga), laughter, tears of joy, utterance of deformed sounds, feelings of fear, the curling back of the tongue, revolving of eyeballs, temporary stopping of breath without effort, an itching or crawling sensation under the skin, and singing with ecstasy and joy.

These cleansing kriyas and exercises may be practiced for many years by those who do not have the fortune to receive Shaktipat initiation. Strangely enough, however, the initiate performs them automatically, guided from within, without study of any external source. On a subtle level, one may experience divine harmonies, the sounds of various instruments or mantras, the taste of divine flavors and the smell of sweet fragrances, or divine lights and colors. One may recall past lives, be poetically inspired, feel drunk with the ecstasy of divine bliss, have frightening dreams, or remain completely silent. During all this, the

138     mind remains filled with joy. On an intellectual level, the hidden meaning behind the scriptures and spiritual texts are revealed. Intuition and psychic powers put one in touch with the Divine, bringing security, peace, and a feeling of unseen guidance and protection.

Thus, when the automatic kriyas take place and the entire being functions under the control of prana, the nervous and glandular systems are nourished and revitalized. This in turn removes disease and prepares the body and mind for higher states of consciousness. The mind, being still, learns an important lesson, that of remaining as objectively aware as possible, increasing its capacity to maintain objectivity as the disciple progresses along the path.

It is important to understand that the manifestation of Shakti, though automatic and involuntary, can be consciously controlled and stopped at any time. The feelings produced and the physical effects are all under objective observation by the mind even during the most intense periods. The mind is subordinate and surrendered as long as the aspirant lets himself go and does not fear. With complete surrender Shakti can purify the mind and body very quickly and effectively. Hence, nothing goes wrong because the Shakti and the Guru psychically protect the disciple. All such manifestations have a cleansing effect, though they may seem terrifying to the outside observer who knows nothing of Kundalini Yoga.

The physical manifestations which occur with the movement of Shakti correspond exactly to the biblical description of the day of the Pentecost: "and suddenly there came a sound from heaven as of a rushing mighty wind, and it filled the house where they were sitting. And there appeared unto them cloven tongues like as of fire and it sat on each of them. And they were all filled with the Holy Spirit and began to speak with other tongues, as the Spirit gave them utterance" (Acts 2:2-4).

Whenever the right conditions are provided, experiences somewhat similar to Shaktipat can be observed, as in the

Pentecostal Church. Others who experience slight varia-
tions of this awakening are those who practice Subud,
Quakers (who were originally called that because they
quaked), and Holy Rollers. It may also manifest itself on the
psychiatrist's couch and in group therapy sessions, or during drug experiences.

However, as soon as the person goes back to his usual
living habits, the impurities and distractions return. Most
of the systems described above lack the program charted by
enlightened masters which leads the aspirant step-by-step
to the highest peaks of spiritual enlightenment. Such experiences, if not properly guided and guarded by the grace of
the Guru, do not serve their real purpose.

### Surrender to Prana

The average person ignores the dictates of the divine
prana's inner guidance. This is because modern man has
allowed his pranic energies to be dissipated indiscrimi-
nately in sense and ego satisfaction. When prana dictates
sleep, man will say, "I'd rather go to the movies." Where
prana gives the signal for elimination, man will respond
after he has finished some work. Thus he ignores and
insults God's power that tries to function for his well-being.
Kundalini awakening reestablishes these natural prompt-
ings and hence the higher natural disciplines become a way
of life in a most effortless manner. After Shaktipat, meditation becomes natural and takes place without strain or
striving. Preoccupation with time and/or physical discom-
fort gives way to joy and ecstasy.

Because man is a creature of habit (the gross karmic
effects of samskaras) he receives impulses from the subconsciously suppressed past. As a result, he finds himself
performing actions and entertaining thoughts and emotions which obviously destroy his peace and keep him on a
merry-go-round of worldly sufferings. His life is sporadi-
cally "fun", but each "up" is always accompanied by a

140    "down" leading to an endless pattern of sorrow, depression, fear, and insecurity.

The best way to come out of this self-created, self-imposed compulsive destruction is to truly and sincerely accept the divine force known as Krishna or Christ. When we regard them as savior and say, "My Lord, Thy will be done, not mine," we can be free in the real sense. With the recognition of the divine prana as the basic energy which sustains the entire universe, we may realize its presence within ourselves. At the awakening of this energy within, man is transformed into superman and he assumes his heritage as a true son of God.

# Shaktipat Kundalini Yoga: Frequently Asked Questions

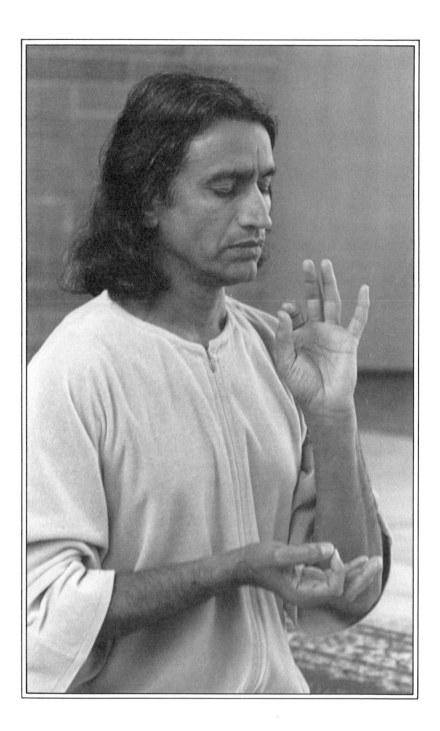

## Kundalini Shakti 143

### What is Kundalini?

Kundalini is the evolutionary energy that lies within each man. In the average individual Kundalini Shakti sleeps at the base of the spine, binding the person to the darkness of ignorance and ego. But when Kundalini awakens it rises through the spine, piercing the six chakras (nerve plexuses) and uniting with Brahman—Cosmic Consciousness—in the seventh, and highest chakra.

Psychologists tell us that the average person is hardly using ten percent of his total capacities. Billions and billions of brain cells are lying dormant. We do not ever use them. When Kundalini awakens, it begins to activate different areas of the body, the nerve centers in the physical body as well as the corresponding centers of consciousness which exist on subtler realms. It begins to effect a definite chemical, biological change in the body. As a result the individual's breath pattern will change. His perceptions will change. Just as a person taking psychedelic drugs can experience the simplest object with sharp intensity, so also when a yogi experiences Kundalini awakening he is able to penetrate into any mystery of nature. New sensitivity, awareness, clarity, imagination, creativity—all these aspects begin to work because this evolutionary energy—this Divine Mother Kundalini Shakti—unfolds each and every layer of man's consciousness and makes it active. Each chakra cleared opens up new layers of understanding, new capacities, new abilities, new dimensions. As a result, any human being can become a genius. Any human being can exhibit superhuman characteristics with this energy.

The energy of Kundalini Shakti has been known to mystics of all religions, but it is only the yogis who have preserved this knowledge and formalized it into a step-by-step method, based on logic and science and suitable to the modern mind.

144     **What is the difference between Prana and Kundalini Shakti?**

Prana is the basic unit of all that you see, all that you feel, all that you experience, all that has a name and a form—everything. It is the primal energy from which everything has emerged. Man is the highest expression of evolution that exists on earth. In his evolutionary journey man has grown by different stages. Prana has been responsible for this entire process of growth. As long as evolution expresses itself in the vegetable or animal kingdoms, it is unconscious. Growth is done directly by nature itself. The consciousness is collective. But as soon as you reach the evolutionary stage of man there is a special consciousness. Man has individual growth because he has been given independent consciousness. The burden of growth is upon him because he has been given free choice. As soon as man comes to the evolutionary level of consciousness, Prana assumes the form of Kundalini Shakti, or Shakti.

Now man has become an individual soul made in the image and likeness of his Father. Now, through the awakening of Kundalini, he has the potential to become one with his Father. So it is Prana, appearing in human beings, which is sleeping at the base of the spine and is known as Kundalini Shakti. The basic unit of Kundalini Shakti is Prana.

**How is Kundalini awakened?**

There are basically three ways of awakening Kundalini. It may awaken accidently and spontaneously, as the result of incomplete spiritual practices of a past lifetime. In such cases, a person unfamiliar with the subject will fail to understand the nature of his experience. Without proper guidance he may become frightened and fail to progress further. Kundalini may also be awakened by various mechanical means, through the practice of Hatha Yoga exercises, breathing techniques, locks and purification methods, through Yamas and Niyamas (mental and moral

disciplines), concentration, meditation, or Mantra Yoga. 145
These are all conscious and mechanical methods. But the
third and highest means of awakening Shakti is through
Shaktipat, the transference of psychic energy by the Master. On coming into the presence of a Guru, the person who
is ready and open begins to feel waves of bliss. He experiences something new, something unusual that he doesn't
understand. But he feels very different. Involuntary motions begin to occur. He may feel heat or cold, sometimes
crying, sometimes laughing or even shaking for no apparent reason. All the while he feels ecstatic. These are some of
the ways by which you can recognize that the Shakti has
been awakened.

The experience of Shaktipat transforms a person's entire attitude toward life. Negative habits of acting and
thinking are removed as he begins to feel progressively
more awakened and opened to love. This love begins to
radiate from him. There is a very deep change in his whole
energy pattern. These changes—this awakening—occurs
by the very look of the Master, the very touch of the
Master, the very word of the Master. It can occur even at a
great distance from the Master. It ultimately results in a
change of the individual's entire lifestyle and personality.
And it is a permanent change.

### How do you give Shaktipat?

My own Gurudev is His Holiness Swami Shri Kripalvanandji Maharaj, who is one of the few living Kundalini
Yoga Masters who has reached the highest state of Nirvi-
kalpa Samadhi after 27 years of unceasing perseverance
and practice. Realizing the present spiritual need in the
West, Gurudev gave me Shaktipat Diksha on January 7,
1969, along with his very rare and special blessings to
transfer this psychic power to my Western disciples.

Since that time thousands of seekers have been guided
to me to receive the grace of Shaktipat. I do not feel that it is

146    I who is giving Shakti. It is not given by my choice nor does it come from me. It is God's divine power that flows through me by the grace of my Divine Master. Those who are ready for it are automatically attracted towards me, love me, and want to be around me. This Shakti responds most to love, Divine love, and surrender. People having these qualities attract Shakti from me. Whenever someone draws Shakti from me I am aware of it, even if the person is behind me or in a large crowd. Thus, Shakti acts as a most sensitive detector of love.

## The Role of the Guru

### What is the role of the Guru in Shaktipat Kundalini Yoga?

During the process of Shaktipat Diksha (Shakti Initiation), the astral body of the Guru merges with that of the disciple, establishing a strong energy contact between the two which guards and protects the disciple. At this time the Master takes on the karma of the initiate, thus speeding up the evolutionary process of the disciple. The same process of karmic ties is expressed in Christianity by the statement that Christ suffered and died for our sins (I Cor. 15:3). Shaktipat initiation creates an astral link between the Guru and disciple by which the disciple continues to receive help from his Guru and the chain of Masters associated with his Guru.

The Yogic scriptures declare that, for the disciple's quickest growth, he should be totally dedicated to the Guru. He should love the Guru, do everything for the Guru, and keep the Guru in his heart all the time. This is a difficult concept for the average Westerner, because in the West you are taught to be on your own, taught to boost your ego, taught to be separate from everyone else. Everything possible is done not to surrender to anyone and to make it on your own. So it is difficult to establish the true Guru-disciple relationship.

In Kundalini Yoga, however, despite such deep-seated

cultural training, a disciple could know nothing about the Guru-disciple relationship, and after receiving Shakti from a Master he will at once feel that his Guru lives within him. It is actually the astral body of his Guru that has come into him because he has received his Guru's energy. When Christ instructed his disciples to take the bread of his flesh and drink the wine of his blood, it symbolized the consuming of his energy—his Shakti. So on this path the Guru's energy actually enters the disciple. From that point the disciple experiences the ecstasy of joy and growth. His Guru's picture, his face, his attitudes, his ways of working, thinking, moving, walking—all will enter the disciple. Immediately this connection between the two will generate a great flow of knowledge. The Guru can then teach without talking to the disciple because the link of love allows the disciple to learn without the struggle usually involved in spiritual practices. Only love can carry what the tongue cannot convey, what language cannot express. The attitude of love is a spontaneous occurrence on this path of yoga.

### What role does the disciple's attitude, desire for growth, and openness play on the path of Shaktipat Kundalini Yoga?

In this area it is not just the Guru who plays a role, it is the disciple as well. If two men go to the river for water, one carrying a cup and the other carrying a bucket, will not one bring back more than the other? It is the disciple's degree of openness which determines how much he is capable of receiving.

They say that when the disciple is ready the Guru will appear. If the disciple is not ready, and the Guru appears physically, it does not mean that the Guru has appeared. The Guru will appear only to that person who establishes a contact of love energy with the Guru. The Guru never inflicts his energy on anyone without the person's cooperation. Not even God will take that privilege. It is said that God helps those who help themselves. It begins with you.

148 The first Guru is within you. God is within you. But to receive His energy you must be ready. You must want it wholeheartedly and you must be open.

Sometimes you may not be consciously aware that you have a true desire for growth. You may doubt your own worthiness to receive from a Guru, or question your ability to be open. On a very deep-seated, unconscious level, however, you have the desire to grow. By remaining receptive, rather than by judging your own worthiness, you will have the necessary openness to receive the grace of the Guru.

**After the inner Shakti has been awakened, is an external Guru still necessary?**

Once the Shakti is awakened the Guru within you also begins to awaken and provide all the guidance necessary for your growth. But in the initial stages, while there are still great impurities of the mind and ego, the inner guidance can also be impure. When the inner Guru leaves the heart and moves to the head, then you need the help of the external Guru.

When Shakti rises you go through a quicker evolutionary process. You purify yourself so fast that you come across more difficulties. But these difficulties are not the same as the problems you previously encountered. When a car is driving at twenty-five miles per hour in the rain, there are so many drops that will hit the windshield within one minute. If the same car is going fifty miles per hour, twice as many rain drops will hit it. Those who progress faster seem to have more difficulties, but these are all part of the purification process. This is the first stage of Kundalini awakening. You may experience disappointments, frustrations, and deep depressions. It will happen because the blocks of many lifetimes are being released. As they go out, they throw their aroma around you. There is nothing to worry about. You are emptying your garbage and so it may smell bad for a while. Fighting this process will only prolong your sense of frustration, but if you surrender you will go through these purifications without difficulty. At this stage the guidance of the Guru is necessary. By yourself you lack the strength to trust, but if you love your Guru enough, you'll be able to trust him. Then your doubts can be removed. A surrounding conducive to growth is especially important at this time. In the Ashram situation you can receive the love and help of those who have already had similar experiences, as well as the support of those going through the same stage. With this support, and by the grace of your Guru, you realize that this is just a cleansing phenomenon.

**It is said that the true Guru is within. Is it necessary to have an external Guru?**

Many people feel that they don't need a Guru. They say, "My Guru is within. I don't need an external Guru." That's a very superficial concept. Because despite their claims to having an inner Guru, most of these people show no signs of personal transformation. They lack the ability to affect a significant change in their lives. Their belief in an inner Guru is not based on their personal experience. It is an intellectual, borrowed, verbal belief.

When you have a Guru within, you have the strength to practice any discipline without flaw, fear, or distraction. In the midst of disturbances you remain as calm and centered as the eye of a cyclone. Whether you have name, fame, and glory or are hated, you remain balanced. When you reach such a state of inner balance and harmony, when you are the same despite raging storms around you, when you are in the world but not of the world, then you have an awakened inner Guru. Then, and only then, can you grow without an external Guru.

What you can do in your Guru's presence is difficult to do in his absence. Can you learn piano without a teacher with the same speed, the same technique, the same refinement that you'd learn in a teacher's presence? It might take you years to learn without a teacher what you could learn in the shortest possible way in the teacher's presence. The spiritual path is much more intricate than learning to play a piano. A Guru is necessary.

### Is it necessary to have one Guru only, or can you learn from several teachers at once?

There was a time when young people collected money, name, fame, and possessions. This was one kind of greed. The youth of today have become disenchanted with this materialism, but they don't know what to replace it with. As a result, they replace material greed with spiritual greed. In this new seeking, which is actually spiritual greed, they collect words and books and Masters and techniques and philosophies. They go from one collection to another and then somehow convince themselves that they are spiritual seekers, but they are not.

Of course, there is a place for this kind of seeking. But there is also a time to settle. There is a time to go out and try different paths, different Gurus, different approaches, so long as it is done with conscious awareness and undertaken as a true search. A search is not a true search unless it is practiced in a concentrated, focused manner. But some people become so habituated to seeking that they escape in the name of seeking. In the name of seeking, in the name of universality of approach, they are becoming distracted.

Unless you eventually come to a very precise, one-pointed direction with one Guru and one approach, a path that you can pour your whole heart into, there is no way you can make it. Those who go from one Guru to another are digging fifty holes five feet deep and expecting to find water. If instead they dug one hole two hundred fifty feet deep, they would definitely discover the water of spiritual truth.

## Does surrender to a Guru mean the loss of individual identity or the sense of caring about your own growth?

By surrendering you do not become careless, but you do become worry-less. This is the true meaning of surrender. Surrender is being in the here and now. It is saying, "My Lord, thy will be done." As soon as you say this, you stop projecting into the future and yet the future is taken care of in a most unique way, in a better way than ever before. You will never make a better future by thinking about the future all the time. This is absurd. As soon as you project into the future, you have fear, you have desire, you have ego, and you don't have surrender. Once you remove the selfish desires from your life as much as you can and surrender to God, there is nothing He can't cure. But He has a price. He says, "Surrender all your worries, all your fears to me." That is all He asks. When you stop worrying about yourself, you will be amazed at how fast things change. By surrendering worries, you are removing the source of all unhappiness, disease, and problems—psychological, emotional, or physiological. There is no other cure that is better than this.

## Why is selfless service to the Guru (Guru Seva or Karma Yoga) so highly recommended?

All the Yogic scriptures say, "Love your Guru. Serve him in every way." The Guru does not need your service. It does not benefit him, but it helps you to grow. When you love someone, you become like him. When you dwell on someone, you are transformed into him. When you meditate constantly upon your Guru through love and selfless service, you establish a channel of energy so that the communications that exist on a higher, subtle level can be established. The system of Guru Seva is both psychological and scientific. When you give a gift to someone, you are more capable of accepting a gift from him. When you help someone, you become more open to his energies. So also

152    when you serve your Guru with love, you increase your capacity to receive what he has to give.

Guru Seva or Karma Yoga is a most effective method of purification. Physical energy, emotional energy, and spiritual energy are all forms of prana. God has given you these energies for right use to help humanity and, through helping, to aid your soul's growth. So every form of work which becomes your lot can serve as an act of liberation from desire, tension, jealousy, hatred, anger, and lust. Thus each act becomes worship when done with love and the spirit of service. Each act becomes a process of cleansing, a way of refining your problems.

Some people only breed further problems when they work. They create hatred by work. They create fear by work. But when you work to serve your Guru you remain non-attached to the results of your actions. You want nothing but to serve, and so you have no reason to fear, no reason to hate. When work is done in this way, with the right attitude of mind, with devotion, with love, your actions become a spontaneous expression of love rather than an expression of fear or competition. Then you are truly serving your Guru, because your Guru is first within you. This is why service to the Guru is service to yourself—your higher self. This service is the true Karma Yoga that destroys all past karma and stops the birth of new karma.

## Meditation

**What meditation technique is recommended in Shaktipat Kundalini Yoga?**

Meditation on the Guru is the most effective means of receiving his grace. The Guru imparts a Mantra (a potent sound formula), teaches the technique of repeating it, and awakens the Shakti within you—consequently meditation on him leads you to the highest goal. Contemplation of the Guru is the very essence of Kundalini Yoga. This contem-

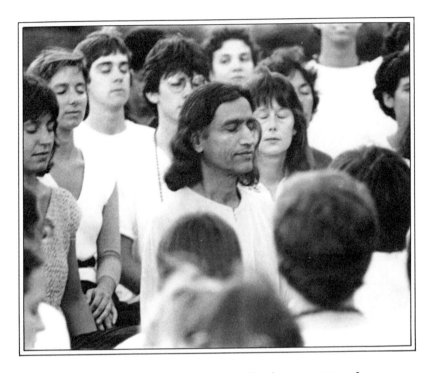

plation goes on within throughout all other activities. It transforms the disciple's life into a continuous meditation. As the disciple constantly remembers his divine Guru, the Guru begins to work within him, washing away all of his impurities and raising his finite being to infinite Godhood.

On the path of Kundalini Yoga when you sit for meditation you surrender. You invoke the presence of your Guru and take his image into your heart. Then you say, "My Lord, take over." Your body may begin to move or it may be still. It may fall down or you may be standing on your head. You could be dancing, you could be laughing, you could be crying. Everything that is done is coming from within. The inner energy knows what is right.

In most meditations you consciously choose one technique. Then you sit right and try to meditate. When you are consciously trying, your mind will constantly feel a disturbance and your body will constantly create a distraction. They will not let you meditate. It's a lot to contend with.

154       In Kundalini Yoga both mind and body are used as assets rather than as distractions. After Shaktipat, the Shakti begins to rise and to create movements automatically. When you sit in meditation and you feel like rocking, you rock, if you feel like crying, you cry, if you feel like jumping, you jump. You witness everything that happens and you feel blissful. Your mind is the observer of everything that is happening to the body and through the body. Your awareness becomes choiceless. Meditation is a spontaneous, effortless occurrence.

## The Manifestations of Shakti

**What types of manifestations are experienced after Shaktipat? What is the purpose of these manifestations?**

      Immediately after receiving Shaktipat the awakened power of Kundalini Shakti begins its work of purifying the entire being. The disciple may soon experience noticeable changes on all levels, physical, mental, emotional, and spiritual. You may be aware of a changed outlook towards life and a more refined perception of spiritual matters. As Shakti becomes more and more fully awakened, it begins to affect both the autonomic nervous system, which functions under pranic intelligence alone, and the voluntary nervous system, which functions under mental control. Under the effect of powerful currents traveling through the entire nervous system, the Shakti assumes its original role as master of the entire being. The voluntary nervous system becomes autonomic for a time, while the mind becomes a mute spectator of the working of this divine inner intelligence. The Shakti, freed from the mind's usual tyrannies, acts as a purifying force wherever necessary within the disciple, creating a variety of physical and spiritual experiences which vary according to the individual's needs and capacities. The disciple might experience heat, cold, involuntary shaking, crying, or laughing from joy, automatic breathing of various kinds, spontaneous yogic asanas, mudras and locks (performed perfectly even without conscious knowledge of Hatha Yoga), dancing and singing in ecstasy, divine visions, smells, sounds, and tastes, voices of inner guidance, memories of past lifetimes, unusual visions and dreams, and the sensation of divine ecstasy. (For accounts of Shakti experiences, see page 168). Throughout all of these experiences the nervous and glandular systems are being nourished and revitalized by the activated Shakti. Disease, mental tensions, and emotional blocks are removed by cathartic methods which bear many similarities to modern psychology's techniques of Gestalt and Primal Therapy. There are many, many complexes which have been stored and suppressed in the subconscious. In the meditation of Kundalini Yoga you surrender your conscious control to the workings of Shakti. As soon as you do this, the top of the bottle is taken off—the subconscious is now open—and the blocks and pent-up energy which have been clouding the sun of your divine soul are removed.

### Can Shakti manifestations be controlled?

Whenever you voluntarily accept anything it is within the realm of your conscious choice to deliberately stop it as well, and so although they are automatic and involuntary, the manifestations of Shakti can be consciously controlled and stopped at any time. The feelings and the physical effects produced are under objective observation by the mind even during the most intense periods. The mind is subordinate and surrendered as long as you let yourself go and do not fear. With complete surrender Shakti can purify the entire being very quickly and effectively. The constant, psychic protection of the Guru guards the disciple who has surrendered himself at all times.

## 156     Is Kundalini Yoga dangerous?

Many writers have described the path of Kundalini Yoga as a dangerous path. The same could be said for learning to drive a car without the supervision of an experienced driver. The safest and easiest method of awakening the Divine Mother Shakti is by the grace of a Master experienced on the path. Even if Shakti is awakened by other methods, the Guru's grace is essential for true progress.

It is recommended that beginning practitioners of Kundalini Yoga limit their time of meditation to two hours a day. Purification is the basis of this path. Because the beginner has not sufficiently purified his ego, mind, emotions, and body, he must work to consciously purify through selfless service, positivity in thought and speech, Hatha Yoga, and control of sensual, selfish desires. Then he may progress more deeply into meditation. Should you find at any time that your manifestations make it difficult to cope with the realities of job and family, immediately reduce your meditation time. You must always retain the ability to function with reason after any manifestation.

Peace of mind is the main thing. Some people do not manifest at all, yet their minds are calm and at peace, while others, who may be manifesting, may not necessarily have the results of peace and harmony. First try to change yourself, your everyday thinking, and patterns of jealousy, hatred, and competition. This basic purification is the key. If you are already manifesting, work on purification. If you don't manifest, work on purification and you will have manifestations. Then even if manifestations never happen, it will be all right because you have already accomplished the one purpose of all manifestations—purification.

Persons having a history of serious emotional disorders should not go too quickly into the stage of Shakti manifestations. For these people further purification of the mind and body is strongly suggested as a preparation for Kundalini Yoga.

## Why do different individuals manifest differently, and others not at all?

We are each an individual combination of many, many things. There is no one person who is exactly like another person, and so there are no two people who will manifest in the same manner for the same length of time. Manifestations are purely personal. Your own personality makeup will determine your response.

# Surrender

### Explain the role of will versus the role of surrender on the path of Shaktipat Kundalini Yoga.

There is only one way you will be able to solve the mystery and the misery of life, and that is by going within. Everything that externalizes your energy causes distractions, distress, and disappointments. In order to go within there are two stages for most people. The first stage is conscious, the second is automatic, spontaneous, natural, and effortless. The first stage requires effort, but almost everyone has to go through it in order to arrive at the second stage. A space ship going to the moon needs propelling power up to the point where gravity becomes nil. At that point the gravity of the opposing planet will suck the ship along. The first stage of this space ship's travel takes effort, but the second stage is effortless.

There are many paths that lead to the path of effortlessness, but they are footpaths. They are paths of the will and they all can vary and change so far as the individual is concerned. But as soon as you arrive at the path of surrender—the effortless path, the pathless path, the path of all paths—then you must give up all your efforts and surrender to the will of the Lord.

So the path that is for one cannot be for all, because each person is a very special individual. The path that is for all cannot be for one, because the path that is for all is a social path, and not a spiritual path. To travel on this spiritual path each person has to travel from the alone to the alone. Although everyone may seem to follow one path, it is just the superstructure of the path that they are following. When you arrive at the path of all paths, the effortless path, the path where the Divine leads you, each person must go through a different avenue, because each one has a different requirement, each one has a different past, each one has a different personality. If any one path is imposed on these different personalities, it becomes a supreme imposition, a strain, a fight.

Everything that I'm teaching is meant to lead you to that effortless path. When Shakti awakens fully, you arrive at that path, the pathless path. This is the only path that can be a universal path. It is the only path that can be the highest path for on it you are not doing anything at all. Nothing that you are doing is done by you, nothing that you are doing is imposed on you, nothing that you are doing from that point on is coming from outside to you, and nothing that you learn has been told to you nor have you read about it. From that point on everything that the Shakti does is precisely designed for your body, mind, emotions, precisely designed to fit what you are at any given moment. This is how meticulously the divine energy does its most careful work to purify you. There is no Guru, there is no medicine man or psychic, there is nobody who exists on this earth who can give you the kind of technique that will be suitable to you to the extent that it changes itself at every moment according to the requirement of your body chemistry, your glandular chemistry, your physiological, mental, and biological state, your expectations, your past, and your future. Everything will fall in place precisely with this divine energy of God which we call Kundalini Shakti. This energy is omnipotent, omniscient, and omnipresent. There is no path that can match this path because it is none of your doing. Now you are following the basic essence of all teachings that have ever been taught on the face of the earth. The highest teaching is, "My Lord, Thy will be done, not mine." But this is possible only when Shakti rises. Otherwise you can exert effort and you can succeed to some extent, but you will have difficulties. So the path of Kundalini Yoga is the pathless path. This is not necessarily so from the very beginning but sometimes it can be. If you awaken Shakti through the conscious methods of Hatha Yoga, Bhakti Yoga, and Mantra Yoga, Kundalini Yoga is a footpath. But as soon as Shakti rises you will arrive at the pathless path, the pathless path that is the true universal path.

**Should all conscious yoga practices be abandoned after receiving Shaktipat?**

In yoga there are two stages of practice. The first stage is consciously doing practices of asanas and pranayama with discipline, method, and technique. You follow practices according to what you have consciously learned. This stage is what I call a footpath. The purpose of the footpath is to lead you to the second stage, which is spontaneous and automatic, which is the pathless path. When Shakti awakens, the purifying movement of prana causes spontaneous kriyas, postures, and breathing. At this stage you have reached the pathless path, which is suited specifically to your personal needs. You surrender and allow the body as well as the breath to move in whatever way it comes from within. In the first stage, the footpath, you should practice consciously and willfully. Those who experience postures and breathing spontaneously and automatically, however, should allow them to happen spontaneously and automatically, without any control of the mind.

## 160   Practical Application

**Why is the practice of celibacy (brahmacharya) tradition-
ally associated with Kundalini Yoga?**

Within this body there are many miracles hidden. The
same force—the same energy—that is used for the sexual
act can be transmuted into energy for higher growth. This
sexual energy is one and the same as Kundalini energy. In
the average person sexual energy is drained and dissipated
with sensual indulgence, but the yogi who knows how to
channel it upwards can transmute the sexual energy into
pure love, lasting growth, and bliss far surpassing any
temporary, sensual experience. This energy is the basis of
everything you want in life. It is the most physical form of
the divine soul—the Atman. And so you must learn how to
guard this energy, how to save it from being misused and
abused. Through observing brahmacharya, you will learn
the proper use of energy. Because sex is the master energy,
by harnessing it you automatically bring all other energies
under control.

**Can a married person progress on this path while main-
taining a normal sex life?**

Celibacy is not one-hundred percent necessary so long
as sex is not abused. Married couples can practice this path,
as can people who are living a regular life of business.

Many married people have reported that their interest
in sex decreased automatically after receiving Shaktipat.
This is because the energies that were formerly channelled
downward through sexual stimulation are now being
transmuted and directed upward for spiritual growth. It is a
natural phenomenon. It is important at this time to remain
sensitive to the needs of the other partner, especially if he
or she is not on the spiritual path. A moderate sex life
within marriage will not be detrimental to your growth.
The decline of interest in sex is neither permanent nor

beyond your conscious control. Since the upward transmutation of energy is only partial, the individual can still channel his energies into sex if he so desires.

There is a stage in Kundalini Yoga, however, where the sexual urge becomes very powerful. As Divine Shakti rejuvenates the entire body, the glands begin to work most quickly and efficiently in producing sexual hormones to aid this rejuvenation process. At this time the guidance of the Guru is absolutely necessary for the aspirant, who must learn the proper methods of raising and channelling this potent energy.

## What is the most effective way to interest a spouse and family in the spiritual life?

By your example. When your loved ones see you becoming kinder, more loving, more considerate of their needs then they will be open to investigating the cause of this change in you. But if you prematurely try to convince them with verbal, intellectual arguments, you will only make them antagonistic to your practices. Frequently one partner in a marriage can use their interest in the spiritual life as an excuse to start an argument in the family. They are not interested in yoga, but in competing with their partner. This is not spiritual growth.

I have seen many times that as one partner becomes interested in yoga the other partner becomes less interested. Should the disinterested spouse begin to become involved the first partner will frequently show a decline of their original interest. This is not a matter of interest but of difficulties that were already present in the relationship. The ego cannot handle the threat of the spouse acquiring a new loyalty. This is why I teach that if a wife is very much interested in growing she should be fully dedicated to her husband. First become a wife and then a yoga student. Of course, the same applies to husbands. This doesn't mean that you can't practice yoga and still love and serve your

162     spouse. You can still practice, but give your partner the priority of your love because the real measure of your growth is the love in your heart.

### Is it necessary to live in an Ashram after receiving Shaktipat?

When Kundalini becomes active it is like a seed given to the disciple. After this seed is planted it has many other needs: it needs sunshine, loving care, showers, and protection. The disciples who receive the seed of Shaktipat should also follow the rules of caring for it. They should find the surrounding that will help them and encourage them to follow a lifestyle conducive to growth. Ashram life provides a setting of support in which these practices of Kundalini Yoga can be carried out with maximum ease. Those whose situation permits should consider living at the Ashram, either temporarily or for an extended period. In this environment the seed of Shakti will quickly grow to a strong tree.

But Ashram life is neither possible nor necessary for those with family commitments or other strong responsibilities. If you can draw upon the presence of your Guru by following his teachings, you will live in the Ashram of all Ashrams, with the Guru of all Gurus.

The following guidelines will help you create an Ashram within your own home:

1.     It is not unusual for doubts and questions to creep in gradually. Discussing your precious personal experience with the wrong people can only confuse you with opinions. You have the choice—whether to accept the opinions of others or your own experience. The mind lives on doubts and opinions. The heart lives on experience. Listen to your heart. Your mind may try to stunt your growth by inventing doubts, fears, imaginary difficulties, and feelings of unworthiness

and inadequacy. Don't believe them. Believe what you have experienced.

2. If you are fortunate enough to be near a group associated with Kripalu Ashram, take advantage of your good fortune. Join your brothers and sisters frequently for support and love. If there is no such group in your area, join with others who have experience to create one. In your unity you will find strength. Company is stronger than willpower. A group will provide the great moral support needed in the early stages of growth. You may call the Ashram for guidance in forming such a group.

3. Command within you the presence of your Gurudev. Visualize him in your meditation and place your questions before him. Guidance will come. Always remember that true love for your Guru is the practice of his guidance and teachings.

4. Plan to visit Kripalu Ashram at least four or five times a year. You will discover that each visit to the Ashram deepens your growth and love. During these visits, you will receive detailed guidance for your daily practices.

5. Eat pure, simple, nourishing, balanced foods. Always eat in moderation. Eat two meals per day. At the third mealtime take milk, fruit, and/or fresh salad. Avoid all stimulants: liquor, coffee, tobacco, drugs, meat, garlic, onions, etc. All unessential medication should also be avoided.

6. Fasting is very important for purification. Fast every Thursday. Every three months, fast for three to five consecutive days for major purification. This period can be increased according to your need and capacity. Fast on one kind of fruit or fruit juice or on water alone. Whenever possible, fasting should be done with silence and a prayerful attitude. Japa should be increased during periods of fasting.

7. Avoid meaningless conversation. Speak the truth pleasantly. Maintain uniformity of thought, word, and action.

8. Reduce your wants to needs. Simplify and purify your life by practicing the Yamas and Niyamas (moral guidelines of ancient India).

9. Practice celibacy or sexual moderation, as your circumstances permit. Practice self-control and moderation in all sensual matters. As with all disciplines, practice awareness rather than abuse, sublimation rather than suppression.

10. Practice yoga asanas, pranayama, and meditation for a minimum of one and a half hours per day, regularly. Learn and practice as many asanas as possible, but do the following daily: shoulderstand, plow, bridge, fish, headstand, yoga mudra, camel, cobra, twist, and abdominal lift. This can be divided between 45 minutes of practice in the morning and 45 minutes in the evening. Include an afternoon practice if possible. Increase the length of practice, gradually, if you are able. Regular practice will increase your alertness, help to control lower desires, and result in quick spiritual progress. Should the automatic movements of Shakti occur during your practices, abandon the conscious exercises and surrender to the workings of Shakti.

11. Always maintain the ability to consciously stop the involuntary manifestations of Shakti at a desired time. You should always be able to function with greater clarity and efficiency as a result of Shakti meditation. Should this become difficult, simply reduce the amount of time spent in meditation. Persons with prior strong emotional disorders should first purify themselves through conscious practice of Hatha Yoga and acts of selfless service and love.

12. Each day briefly read from the scriptures, such as the **Bhagavad Gita** or the **Bible,** or from other inspiring

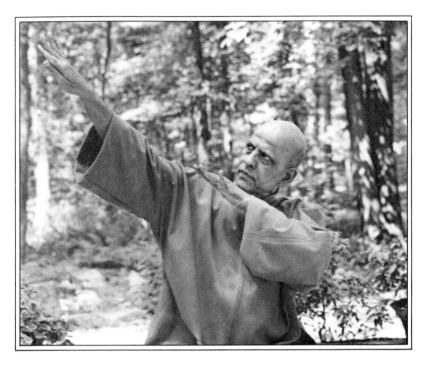

books. Read slowly and reflect deeply on what you have read. I particularly recommend the study of the **Bhagavad Gita,** Chapters 12, 15, and 16, and Shlokas 54 to 72 of Chapter 2.

13. Go to sleep early and rise early. Adjust your sleeping to your individual needs, but maintain a regular schedule. Suggested schedule: sleep by 10:00 pm and up by 5:00 am.

14. Maintain cleanliness and purity of body, both internally and externally.

15. Practice non-violence. Avoid all violent thoughts and words, as well as actions. Non-violence must also include gentleness to one's own self.

16. Maintain awareness, equanimity, patience, and contentment at all times, especially in time of trials.

17. See God everywhere and in everything and act accordingly. Gurudev says, "I bow with reverence to the

many images of the one eternal God. All religions of the world lead to the pious feet of God. So to disrespect any religion, saint, or scripture is great insult to Him."

18. Do not, however, distract yourself from the path in the name of freedom and love for all other paths. Do not indulge in intellectual prostitution. Follow one path which, in time, will lead to a true and direct realization of the unity of all.

19. Perform all actions with awareness and devotion, but with no expectations or attachments to the results. Give help and service whenever the opportunity arises. Serve everyone, particularly your Guru and guru brothers and sisters. Remember that charity begins at home.

20. Earn by honest work and give with an open heart. Donate about 10% without expectation of recognition or reward.

21. Serve and love your Guru in each thought, word, and action. Be always in active surrender to Guru and God. Say, "Thy will be done, not mine."

### What is the purpose of Ashram life?

After the Shakti has been received, many disciplines are required to keep its evolutionary energy active so it can accomplish its task of reaching the highest level of consciousness. It is difficult to follow these disciplines alone. The purpose of Kripalu Ashram is to provide a setting of support in which the practices of Kundalini Yoga can be carried out with maximum ease.

A great yogi once said that company is stronger than willpower. At the Ashram the group's support as well as the continued guidance of the Guru makes the path as effortless as possible. For this reason our Ashram population is steady, except for the constant stream of newcomers, whom we always welcome. Few people leave because they find in this path a fulfillment that satisfies their deepest longings for love and growth. Our disciplines would appear to be strenuous to outsiders yet here these disciplines are the very source of our joy—they are practiced with understanding, love, and support, and this is what makes them work. We keep regular hours, rising daily at 4:00 am and going to sleep by 9:30 pm. Everyone practices Hatha Yoga postures, breathing exercises, and follows a moderate vegetarian diet. We meet for satsanga—chanting and discussion—twice a day. Except for the Ashram staff everyone holds a full-time job outside the community. After work and on weekends they help with various chores around the Ashram. The purpose of all of these practices is to cleanse the disciple on every level—to purify his body, mind, emotions and ego, to strengthen his nerves and awaken love within his heart. This purification is essential to progress on the path of Kundalini Yoga.

**What steps can deepen one's commitment to the path of Shaktipat Kundalini Yoga?**

As these teachings take root in your life, it is natural to desire a deeper commitment to spiritual growth. After three months of sincere practice, you may request Mantra Initiation. At this time, the Guru imparts a mantra (a power-packed spiritual formula) to the disciple, establishing between them a psychic link which continuously provides unseen guidance and protection as it enhances the initiate's spiritual progress.

You will deepen your growth most easily by keeping in close contact with these teachings through visits to Kripalu Ashram, and by attending seminars conducted in many areas of the country by myself and my close disciples. These seminars are a unique opportunity to receive the compact, intensive teachings of Shaktipat Kundalini Yoga.

Concentrate on truly practicing the teachings of one path. Follow the path that transcends all manmade limitations of race, religion, and nationality. Believe in one God manifested through various paths, religions, and masters. At the same time practice only one path in order to truly and deeply experience the underlying unity of all teachings. In the initial stage of spiritual growth too many approaches lead only to confusion. Once you feel a strong bond with a particular Guru, practice his teachings for a sufficient length of time to judge their effects.

## Shakti Experiences

*From hundreds of documented experiences of the manifestations of Shakti, we have chosen from our files a few representations. The divine experiences on these pages occurred by the grace of Shaktipat through the guidance of Yogi Amrit Desai.*

After the first full day of the seminar, as I began to prepare for sleep, I felt an exhilaration of my spirits. I dismissed it as not having "quieted down" from the hustle and bustle of the day. I lay down welcoming the calm and stillness of sleep but, to my surprise, I felt no need for rest or sleep. I felt as though every atom and cell of my body had been activated—instructed to "come alive". Suddenly, there was an urge to run and fly as though I had the wings of an eagle. I wanted to sing and dance through the streets shouting, "I am alive! God is real and alive, and I am filled with God-love!"

Suddenly my mind came tumbling back to the present and rationality. I experienced waves of doubt and fear. Was I losing my mind?

As I lay there, two eyes began to invade my inner vision. Quickly my own eyes opened in disbelief and fright, but the eyes in front of mine did not disappear. The eyes at first seemed to belong to no one, but gradually assumed their proper place on a face. It was your (Yogi Desai's) face. I was startled and disoriented for a brief moment. Then I felt your presence there beside me and the fear disappeared. I fell into a state of consciousness I had been attempting to reach for two years through meditation, the study of books, trying various techniques, and now, having been in your presence for a little more than twenty-four hours, I WAS THERE! Willingly, I submitted to this condition of total relaxation, tranquility, and peace.

Feeling rejuvenated, as though I had slept the entire night, I returned to the seminar in time for morning chanting and meditation. I began to fall into the rhythmic beat of the instruments and chant. I was content until, suddenly, your voice was the only voice and its utterance pierced through each cell of my body, which dared to awaken and dance in subtle vibration of response. Then an intense conflict between my rational mind and a higher power began until a force greater than my conscious will seemed to invade my being and fill each cell with energy. A deep concentration fell upon me and my whole body and mind became fixed upon you. My eyes would not be moved away from you. It seemed as though my consciousness would lead my body into realms of pure bliss only to be challenged and pulled back by my reluctant mind.

The length of time I cannot tell, for I could no longer perceive time or those forms around me. A power seemed to emanate from your essence to me, surrounding my being, engulfing me. Light appeared, encircling your body. I saw you arise (although I knew you had not physically moved) and walk over to me. I then experienced a strange phenomenon. It seemed as though you entered my body and I could no longer resist the power of that overwhelming love. I was familiar with that love—somewhere, I had experienced it before. It was divine—God-love. I surrendered.

Immediately a vibrational force seemed to invade my being, my eyes became focused upon the area between my

170      eyebrows. You touched my forehead and my mind at first resisted, then my whole body and mind focused on that spot and I became that place which you touched. The energy seemed to soar through my body from the touch of your hands. I could not breathe enough of the prana. My breath became heavier, more forceful, and I wanted to fill each minute cell with the "life force". Then came a feeling of complete relaxation and total surrender. I'm afraid I can't remember much more except a feeling of deep love and devotion, and a sense of humbleness, while at the same time elation, bliss, and joy.     S.H.

Columbus, Ohio

It was on a weekend seminar at the Ashram that I finally found myself able to surrender control to the power of Shakti. It was a split: my eyes were closed, and I was calmly observing myself, awe-struck and totally observant, going through the strangest and most violent emotions of my life. The "greatest show on earth" was going on right inside myself, and I was both the spectator and the performer at the same time.

I was marvelling at the way the Shakti power worked its way intelligently through my nervous system, working on areas which particularly need to be worked on in my particular case. I know now what the "Primal Scream" is about, what years of painstaking Gestalt therapy are about: in the flash of a second, at the flick of a finger, my psychic entity seemed to work through hundreds of years of bad karma, scores of pent-up frustrations, burning up miles and miles of closed-loop tapes created in my childhood.

I have seen powerful therapy taking place in Gestalt and Primal settings. I am convinced that Amritji's way of Shakti unfoldment is a hundred times more powerful. I have seen the candidates of the "Primal Scream" trying and trying and trying to scream. On the other hand, with Shakti one does not try, one merely waits for "it" to happen, and when "it" happens, the Shakti itself chooses which form to take out of hundreds of possible forms. Screaming is only one of them.

A.T.
Ontario, Canada

We went into meditation. You (Yogi Desai) began to direct the energy through our bodies and through the chakras. I felt the energy rising. My blood began to vibrate and quiver. I could see the energy rising up through my body as though I were an observer—I was looking down and through my body. I could see the centers becoming more and more active, and growing and pulsating, but then I lost the sight. I became enveloped in light. I traveled up the stream through myself. My fingers became prickly and I was aware of each cell in them. They were moving wildly. I had to shake my hands. The energy pulled my body into a sitting position with no effort on my part. My hands put themselves on my knees in a final surrender. My personality disappeared.

You came over and touched my forehead. It felt as though you were pressing harder and harder, and then the touch went through my head. The light and love and truth touched my very essence. It was like a shock shooting through me.

At this point I could hold on no longer. All was let loose—my breathing, the movement of my body, the light, the love—all was integrated. Off and on, I was aware of what my body was doing. At one point, I realized that my back was arched back so far that my head almost touched the ground. I had reached a state of ecstasy. There was no separation between anything. Love was bright and truth was all.

S.N.
Washington, D.C.

I started to cry and tears came rushing up, and my feet began to shake uncontrollably. A rush of force or power

172 shook me from the bottom up, threw me down on the floor, and made me shake, cry, and tremble all over. It was like a tremendous electrical force filling my body, every cell exploding into golden-white light. I felt the power so great, that the body could not contain it, it just shattered it. When the crying and shaking slowed down, I knew my whole body was different. Every nerve end seemed to have been stretched and expanded, a whole network inside of me was radiating light, at first light with tremendous power and spark, which gradually changed into a softer feeling of golden light.

With this new light inside of me came a total peace and a new feeling of energy, different than I have ever felt before.

I feel that a new freedom is inside of me, as if some bondage has been shattered, blocks removed, and a new being is emerging . . . almost like the butterfly shedding its cocoon.

J.N.
Grand Rapids, Mich.

The first time I saw Yogi Desai, I was attending a yoga convocation at the Watson Homestead Retreat. My eyes were immediately drawn to him, and never left him. I was compelled to watch every move he made, to absorb every word he said. We were led in a program of meditation and as soon as I closed my eyes, my breathing became deep and my body locked itself into the lotus position. The energy flooded my body with such a force; every cell felt like it was exploding.

I was transfixed by his presence and went into deep meditation. Tears were running down my face, and my whole being: body, soul, and mind were flooded with extreme bliss. Never before had I experienced such a feeling of total satisfaction, total expression, total being. There are no words to express it. A woman came over to me and kissed me saying I was just beaming so much joy.

When Yogi Desai began to leave the room, I panicked, because I wanted him to look at me just once for I knew I had found my Guru, my God. So intensely was I feeling, that I could not move. I could not speak, I could not think. All I could do was look at him hoping with every inch of my soul to see his eyes. And then it happened. Just as I thought he had not noticed me, because many people were crowding around him, he looked at me. Could I ever describe how he looked at me? Never. It went straight through me into every inch of my body, and I shut my eyes to keep it there. I began to tremble and my breathing was involuntary. My whole body shook with prana and love, oh, so much love. I could not stand to fight at all. And all the time I knew he was there. I prayed that he would not leave me alone, that he would be there when I opened my eyes. My body filled with intense heat. The prana rushed through my head, filling me with bliss.

From that moment on, I was not aware of time, food, drink. Nothing but this new consciousness. I can't even remember walking or touching the ground. I was aware that my posture was extremely comfortable and erect, that I felt as I was doing a beautiful ballet. I was fascinated by my own movements. And everywhere I looked, I saw light and God and love. There was nothing I didn't conceive, there was nothing I didn't know. I was aware of everyone and everything around me in 360 degrees, and yet my eyes were closed in meditation. I remember once sitting across from Yogi Desai, and as I looked at him a brilliant light spread across his face so intense I had to shut my eyes . . . bliss.

Later, when I was recalling this, I thought perhaps it was just the sun shining in his face, but then I remembered his back was to the windows.

E.P.
Los Angeles, Calif.

.

# Instant Cosmic Consciousness?[1]

## By D. R. Butler[2]

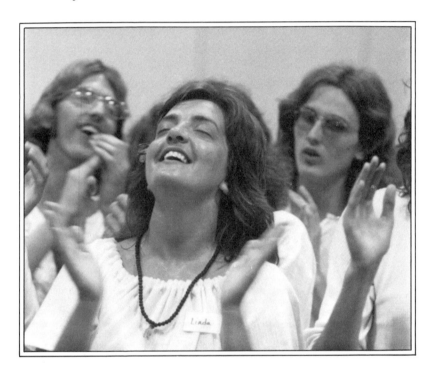

[1] Also appeared in: **Kundalini, Evolution and Enlightenment,** John White (ed.), (New York: Anchor, 1979). Reprinted courtesy of **FATE** magazine.

[2] D. R. Butler is an American yogi who devotes full time to students of his correspondence course in Siddha Yoga. He is a disciple of Swami Muktananda and lives in Forest Hills, New York, where he directs the Queens Siddha Yoga Meditation Center.

176  Instant cosmic consciousness? Well, not really, but it seemed that way for most of the two hundred persons gathered for a week of camaraderie and intense yogic work at Watson Homestead near Corning, New York, for the 1973 ICSA Yoga Convocation (International Center for Self-Analysis in North Syracuse, New York). At that time my wife Pat and I, both in our mid-twenties, had studied yoga for five years. The convocation was an opportunity to devote an entire week to yogic disciplines and to associate with kindred souls.

The first two days were spent with ICSA director Margaret Coble who talked of the Divine Self within us all and told us that the primary goal for the week was to contact this inner self.

For the next three days Roy Eugene Davis, former student of Paramahansa Yogananda and head of the Center for Spiritual Awareness of Lakemont, Georgia, gave us intense instruction in Raja Yoga (meditation and mind control).

Then on Friday morning an unannounced guest arrived. He was Yogi Amrit Desai, a yoga teacher from Philadelphia of whom most of us had never heard. That afternoon, after summing up the various meditation techniques, Roy took a seat behind us on the floor and Yogi Desai went up front to speak or lead chants or do whatever was his "thing". We didn't know.

Clad in a flowing white robe and sitting on the table before us, Amrit easily assumed the lotus posture, his body perfectly poised. He is a handsome East Indian in his late thirties with long black hair and intense dark eyes. He is younger than most yoga teachers but I soon learned he had unusual powers.

He led us into meditation, which is not unusual. Most yoga teachers begin with a meditation. Some chants in Sanskrit followed; still par for the course. I had my eyes closed and I felt pleasant currents of inner energy. Then, as Amrit led us deeper into meditation, I began to realize that something unusual was happening to me.

The first thing I noticed was a wave of euphoria softly permeating my being. I felt intensely happy. I didn't know the reason for the wonderful feeling but I determined to relax and enjoy it.

Suddenly surges of energy—like electrical charges—streaked up my spine. These gradually evolved into a steady current of hot energy flowing from the tip of my spine to the top of my head. My impulse was to analyze intellectually what was happening but I quickly realized that the more I thought about it the less I felt it. So I stopped thinking and concentrated on *experiencing*.

Brilliant colors swirled inside my head; I thought I would burst with happiness. Nothing ever had felt so good! Suddenly a scream burst from someone in the back of the room, then another. In a few moments the place was a madhouse. People were crying hysterically, laughing uncontrollably, gasping for breath, even rolling on the floor. Apparently everyone was experiencing some manifestation of the same energy I was feeling.

I looked at Pat and saw tears rolling down her cheeks. When our eyes met, I knew we both were feeling the same. I closed my eyes and tried to resume meditation—or to experience as intensely as possible whatever was happening. I heard Roy Eugene Davis behind me reassuring various individuals, explaining that he had experienced similar feelings with Yogananda.

Suddenly the whole thing stopped as abruptly as it had begun. The energy inside me subsided and the room quieted. Amrit began to explain what had happened.

We had just undergone what is known as a Shaktipat initiation, he said. This is the awakening of the Shakti or Kundalini which in yoga is the primordial life force, the individualized expression of the Infinite which lies as dormant energy within each of us. The full awakening of Shakti brings about cosmic consciousness; it is experienced physically as total bliss and serenity.

178     All forms of yoga and consciousness development aim at eventually awakening the Kundalini force, but in Shaktipat it happens immediately and spontaneously. The psychic energy is transferred directly from Guru to disciple. Simply by being in Yogi Desai's presence we all had experienced to some degree the awakening of Shakti. How this comes about is somewhat mysterious. Yogi Desai explains that the astral body of the Guru merges with that of the disciple; he also told us that the power came through him from his own master in India (Yogi Desai's Guru is Swami Kripalvananda).

I know that the person who is sufficiently developed to express himself on a certain energy level can cause a manifestation of that same level of energy in another. It might be called a manifestation of mind power—Yogi Desai *thought* and *knew* that the Shakti in the group would be aroused and his concentration was so pure that it was.

Now that the room was quiet Yogi Desai explained that the ostensibly unpleasant manifestations some persons had experienced represented the cleansing of physical, emotional, and psychic impurities. Thus some had screamed and gone into hysterics when subconscious veils were lifted and they had experienced their true natures for the first time. Many persons later confirmed this, reporting that their experiences were ecstatic within, even if they had appeared to be suffering. Many also said that when it was all over they never had felt better in their lives.

Yogi Desai then announced that anyone who wished to leave could do so. More than half of the gathering departed, many obviously shaken by what they could not understand. The rest of us stayed, wanting more.

When there remained only those who wanted to be with him Yogi Desai seemed to radiate even more intense energy than before. My body filled with a brilliant white light and I allowed myself to be absorbed in it. I felt that my life as I previously had known it literally came to an end. My ego identity became meaningless; there was no time; past and future did not exist. All that existed was pure light and pure bliss. I was content to remain in this state forever. When I opened my eyes again I noticed that my body had bent forward; my forehead was touching the floor. I do not remember assuming that position. I was actually bowing down to Yogi Desai! I had never bowed to anyone in my life but some inner unknown force had prompted me—and I knew I wasn't bowing to Amrit Desai the person, but rather to my own higher self which he had helped me see.

He was surrounded by persons who only two hours before had never seen him but now sat on the floor around him, holding his feet, even kissing his feet, weeping unashamedly. Men and women of all ages and professions had found a part of themselves they never knew existed. I knew those people were feeling love and bliss and that Amrit himself was without ego. After a lifetime of practicing intense yogic disciplines he knew he was only a channel for transmitting the energy the others experienced.

At this point someone came into the room and announced it was time to eat. We all laughed uproariously, for food was the furthest thing from our minds. Who would consider leaving such newfound sublimity to put food in his belly? I was willing to leave my body forever if I only could retain that bliss.

Well, Amrit explained, there was more where that came from and we really should eat. My feeling of euphoria continued for several hours, however, and I knew I would never be quite the same again.

I wonder what would happen if those who turn to drugs for glimpses of higher states of consciousness knew that the natural awakening of inner energies through yoga ultimately offers all they are seeking and much more. I wonder what would happen if all our political and religious leaders could spend only an hour or so with such advanced yogis as Amrit Desai. What changes would come over them and what wonders would they perform for the world?

# Gurudev

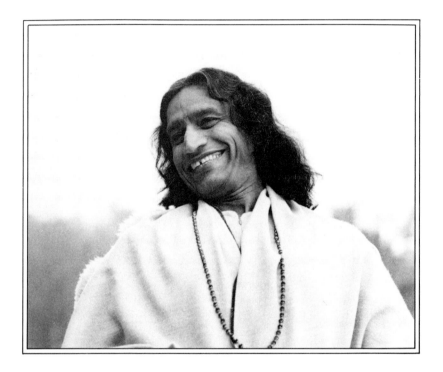

As an expression of deep respect and affection, many people address Yogi Amrit Desai as Gurudev, meaning "beloved teacher". Gurudev is an internationally acclaimed teacher and authority on the ancient science of yoga. He has developed Kripalu Yoga as "meditation in motion", an approach which brings the practice of yoga back to its original depth and dimension.

In 1966, Gurudev founded the Yoga Society of Pennsylvania, which became one of the largest yoga training organizations in the United States. In 1971, he established Kripalu Yoga Ashram, a residential spiritual community and educational organization. It has since become Kripalu

182    Center, the largest residential center for yoga and holistic health on the east coast.

Gurudev has been recognized worldwide and been given many awards and honorary degrees. Chief among these are: Doctor of Yoga Science, given by His Holiness Jagadguru Shankaracharya, one of the leading spiritual authorities of India; Acharya Pravarsha (Supreme Spiritual Teacher), awarded by Swami Vedavyasanandji, Chancellor of Rishikul Sanskrit University; Yogacharya (Spiritual Preceptor), conferred by His Holiness Swami Shri Kripalvanandji.

Lecturing in North America, Europe and India, Gurudev is widely respected for his ability to translate the ancient principles of yoga into a modern format. Both in his discourses and in his several books, he presents a wide range of subjects and incorporates the principles of yoga, psychology and current self-development techniques in a manner easily grasped and practiced in the West, without sacrificing their depth. His teachings are easily understood because they are the direct expression of his experience of life. Infusing both ancient and modern approaches to personal growth with penetrating spiritual insight, Gurudev gives practical tools for applying them for greater health, well-being and spiritual attunement in daily life.

# About Kripalu Center

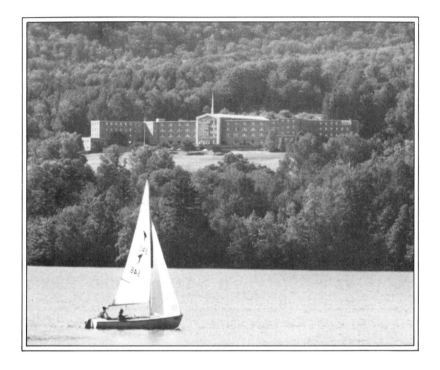

Located among the Berkshire mountains of western Massachusetts, Kripalu Center offers a variety of health holidays, educational programs and individual health services throughout the year. Our 200-member residential staff provides a setting which is uniquely supportive for bringing body, mind and spirit into the balance that is true health.

The basis of our approach is the ancient tradition of yoga and its principle that physical health is the foundation for emotional and spiritual development. Our programs and services combine time-tested yoga practices with more recently developed techniques in holistic health. They each provide experiential learning and first-hand knowledge of

184    vibrant, comprehensive well-being along with practical
methods for living a health-enhancing lifestyle at home.
Weekend, week-long and four-week programs focus
on self-development through yoga, stress management,
fitness, bodywork training and spiritual attunement. Our
programs are excellent both for health professionals who
want to expand the scope of their services and for individuals who, no matter what their background or occupation,
want to derive more satisfaction and joy from their lives.
Our guests can also individualize their visit, choosing from
a wide range of classes, activities and facilities such as
sauna, whirlpool, flotation tank and lakefront swimming.